# THICK BONES

*Causes of and Cures for*

# TEEN OBESITY

Dr. Carol A. Brown

LORAC BOOKS

Boston

# LORAC BOOKS

Published by the Lorac Publishing House, Inc.

64 Forest Street, Boston, Massachusetts 02119

While the author has made every effort to provide accurate telephone numbers and Internet addresses at the time of publication, neither the publisher nor the author assume any responsibility for errors, or for changes that occur after publication.

Copyright© 2010 by Dr. Carol A. Brown

Cover Design © 2010

Chapter Illustrations © 2010

Illustrator Stan Jaskiel

ISBN: 978-1-937649-00-5

Library of Congress Control Number: 2011960423

1. Brown, Carol. 2. Massachusetts—Boston—Fiction.
3. Teen Obesity—Fiction 4. Multicultural—Education

PUBLISHER'S NOTE

This book is a work of fiction. Name, characters, places, and incidents are either the product of the author's imagination or used fictitiously, and any resemblance to actual persons, living or dead, events, or locales is entirely coincidental.

**Manufactured in the United States of America**

# ACKNOWLEDGEMENTS

I want to thank God, who inspired me to write this book and to be a voice for overweight and obese teens. Much thanks to my mom, Mrs. Hanson Brown, who provided me with numerous stories of how her generation prevented obesity, back in the day.

Other family members I'd like to thank include my daughter Tiana Brown, for continued support, my granddaughter Davanna Oliveira, who allowed me to use her name as the main character; Wendy Arthur and nephews Wyndel and Joshua, who provided generational perspectives. In addition, thanks to Ella Robertson, who encouraged me to write a book, and Jane Manning for being my sounding board.

Special thanks to Mrs. Michelle Obama, who brought the issue of childhood obesity to the forefront through her Let's Move Program. Finally, thanks to Ms. Oprah Winfrey, who has continuously brought the issue of obesity to the public's attention.

# CONTENTS

# LIST OF CHARACTERS

DAVANNA BROWN is a fourteen-year-old ninth grader at Cedar Grove High School. Davanna lives in the suburbs with her mom, dad, and her older brother. She is beautiful, confident, a leader, and is thick-boned.

MARITZA RODRIGUEZ is fifteen and in the tenth grade at Cedar Grove High. Maritza used to live in the suburbs before her parents got divorced. Now, Maritza lives in the city with her mom and spends weekends with her dad. She also loves Uncle Jose, her mom's brother. She is gorgeous, humorous, and overweight.

SETH BERNSTEIN is fifteen and a tenth grader along with Maritza. He lives with his mom and dad outside of the city. Seth is sarcastic, smart, and somewhat round.

JOHN WONG is fourteen and in the ninth grade with Davanna. He lives in the city with his dad. It's just the two of them because John's mom died when he was ten. John is brainy, shy, and chunky.

# CHAPTER ONE

## At the Beach

It was a blazing hot, humid, summer day. There was not a cloud in the deep blue sky. Davanna Brown strolled across the beach to meet her friends. She wore a well-fitting orange one-piece bathing suit. Her curvaceous cinnamon hips swayed in the summer breeze. As she passed a group of guys lying on a colorful beach blanket, she could feel them noticing the amount of sensuous junk in her large trunk. With each shift of her sought-after hips, the guys' eyes and bodies stood at attention as if to say, "Damn, I would give anything to get with her."

Davanna didn't stop walking. Her newly manicured toes seeped into the blazing sand. She was gorgeous, with gold-nugget eyes, a big-time attitude, curly brown hair, and thick bones. Her confident body language screamed out, "Stop and look everyone, Davanna has arrived!" She strolled along the beach until she reached her best friend Maritza Rodriguez, who was stretched out on a large blue-and-white beach towel. Maritza was wearing dark sunglasses and a royal blue skirt bathing suit. As she lay on her back, the sun toasted her caramel skin.

Maritza was a funny beauty with long black shiny hair, busty boobs, and thunder thighs. Everyone loved her because she knew how to make people laugh. And when she blinked her black pearly eyes, they could put you into a trance.

"What's up Maritza, long time no sees," Davanna said.

"What's up with you," replied Maritza.

"I can see you're getting your tan on. Girl, your new skin color is hot."

"Thanks! Now, sit down and talk to me."

When Davanna bent over to lay her towel on the hot, grainy sand, even the huge waves at the beach almost stopped to view her cinnamon bottom. When there were no more wrinkles in her orange-and-cream beach towel, she lay down. Face-to-face, the two girls talked and gossiped as they waited for their friends Seth and John, who had volunteered to bring food and drinks. All four teens went to Cedar Grove High School, which was a magnet school that allowed students from other communities to attend. At Cedar Grove, a lot of classes focused on science, technology, engineering, and mathematics.

The boys arrived with the cooler an hour later, just when the girls were getting hungry.

"What took y'all so long?" asked Davanna.

"What do you mean? Did you forget that time stopped until I arrived?" Seth answered.

Davanna just looked at Seth and shook her head. "You are unbelievable."

Seth Bernstein was smart but sarcastic. He believed he knew everything. If you said the moon was blue, Seth would say, "Nah, its aqua." Then he'd explain why it was more aqua than blue. A lot of girls thought Seth was drop-dead gorgeous. He was pale with dark brown curly hair and thick eyebrows. Seth was so full of himself that he was sure he was the finest guy around. He forgot that he was round, with a large jelly roll of stomach that hung over his black-and-white striped swimming trunks.

Seth and John parked the cooler on the beach.

"Y'all look so relaxed," said John.

"Well, have a seat and relax with us." Davanna smiled at her classmate.

John Wong spread his towel next to her. He was shy but self-assured. Even though he kept to himself, he spent a lot of time chatting with his friends online. He was a regular ole computer geek and could solve any technical problem. He was handsome with olive skin, almond-shaped eyes, and straight black hair. Tall but heavyset, he had love handles all the way from his chest to waist.

Seth laid down his towel too, and the four friends talked, cracked jokes, and ate snacks. Though their personalities were different, they had some important things in common: they were all smart, attractive, fun to be around, and overweight.

3

Maritza was funny as hell. She told the others a joke that made them laugh hysterically, so much that they rolled off of their towels onto the sand. They were still giggling when they heard a loud voice behind them.

"Look at those fat asses," it said.

The four friends' laughter immediately turned to silence. The beach got so quiet that they could have heard a bird flying over their heads pass gas.

Davanna slowly looked around to see who had spoken. A tall thin girl wearing a hot red bikini stood down by the water, staring up at them. She held hands with her muscle-man boyfriend who sported tight gold swimming trunks.

Davanna sat up. The words heated her up so much she could have fried an egg on her head. She did not believe that the couple had just sworn at them. She pointed her finger in the air and yelled, "Oh no they didn't! Did y'all hear what they said? They just swore at us!" Her face scrunched up with disgust and her nose twisted like she smelled a skunk.

Red Bikini and Muscle Man turned away and continued walking down the beach.

"But for what? See y'all, they forced it! They must've had a problem with us, because we laughed and looked good. No one else on the beach was bothered when we laughed out loud. I can't get over this. That fake couple really swore at us! They're so fake that girl must have breast implants, and her man is pumped up on steroids."

The others laughed.

But Davanna yelled, "Oh hell no, it's about to be on and popping!"

She got on her feet ready to run toward them, but her friends grabbed her and sat her back down.

She shrugged off their hands and yelled, "Hey you two, I got your fat asses alright. And I'm going to give you a piece of mine!" She wanted a piece of that couple's butts so bad she could taste it.

Her friends held her back from getting up again. They had to wrestle her down on the sand.

"Davanna, stop!" John said. "It's not worth it. Are you going to jump on their butts over a swear?"

"C'mon, don't get so heated! It was just one swear," Maritza told her friend. "Look at them. They're so skinny they look like two crack heads! Remember Davanna, only a dog wants a bone!" Maritza was yelling. She looked so serious that the others laughed at her expression.

"No, it makes me mad," Davanna said. "They don't know us but they think they can judge us. All they looked at was our size. All kinds of people have said and done mean things to me, because I'm overweight. Hasn't that happened to y'all?"

"Of course," John muttered.

Davanna looked around at each of her friends. "You know what? Could I tell y'all some of the things people have said and done? I think it would help me if I talked to my friends about it. I could get all of the negative stuff off my chest. Maybe you've had some of the same experiences. Like somebody used the same insulting gesture as they did to me. Or used the same words."

"I'd like to do that," Maritza replied. "The world would be a better place to live if people wouldn't make fun of me because of my size."

"Yeah, there'd be less hurt feelings and fights, if people would just mind their own damn business," Seth added.

"They don't understand how much I hurt," Davanna said. "That's how I got overweight. I've been through some rough stuff. I'm stronger because of it. But nobody sees that. If people just got to know us, they would see my confidence, Seth's smart sarcasm, Maritza's sense of humor, and John's deep analytical thought process. We all have gifts."

"Don't forget Davanna, we are all fine as hell!" Maritza chuckled.

Davanna lay back and looked out at the beautiful pink-and-orange horizon. "It's a beautiful day. The sky is calm, the water's blue, and I can see the heat waves rise up from the sand. It was so peaceful before."

She lay for a while in deep thought, and so did the others.

"Hey guys." Davanna sat up. "I've never talked to anyone about all the negative things that happen when you're overweight. And we haven't even talked to each other about them.""You know, you're right," John replied.

"Well, I can't see a better time than now. Let's start with the rude encounter from the couple who just swore at us, since we all just experienced it. What do y'all think?"

"Let's go for it, girl!" cheered Seth.

"I agree," Maritza replied.

"I'm with you, Davanna. Why don't you go first," said John.

"Great! Y'all know I don't have a problem going first." And Davanna began her story.

# CHAPTER TWO

## Being Teased or Bullied

"Hi, it's me, Davanna Brown. I'm fourteen. I'm in the ninth grade at Cedar Grove High School. I'm African-American and I live in the suburbs with my mom, my dad, and my eighteen-year-old brother, who is a royal pain in the butt. I'm beautiful, I'm confident, and I'm a leader who also happens to be thick-boned."

Davanna paused for a second.

"Well, I'll talk about a few negative things that happened to me. Okay, that rude couple, who swore at us? They were lucky I couldn't get to them. I was going to beat them, like I beat an egg before I cook."

Davanna sat up on her beach towel and closed her eyes. Her elbows rested on her knees and her hands on her temples. After sitting like that for a while, she ran her fingers through her soft curly hair, shook her head from left to right, and whispered, "I just don't know, I just don't know.

"When you are overweight, people forget you have feelings! You're viewed as a large piece of flesh, with bones but

8

no heart or feelings. But we're not hollow like a turtle that's left its shell.

"I remember the first day of middle school. All of my teachers were great! My classes and schedule seemed easy. The day went fine, until lunchtime. The experience was so awful there that it was the first and last time I ate lunch in the school cafeteria."

"What happened?" asked John.

"As I ate my pizza and fries, kids watched me as if I was some kind of alien. Each time I took a bite of my food, they made animal sounds like *oink* and *moo*. The students who didn't do that made jokes. One student asked, 'What did the fat kid stick you up for?' And somebody else responded, 'Ooh I know, I know, the fat kid stuck me up for my groceries.' Everyone at the table laughed.

"Another student said, 'Fat kids don't run for student government. The only thing they run for at school is lunch.' People laughed until tears fell from their eyes. Then they went right back and made animal sounds, followed by more jokes.

"As I sat there, my blood boiled. I was heated. I had had enough. This time y'all weren't there to hold me back, like you did today. I put both of my hands on the lunch table and pushed up from my seat. I walked over to the group of students with major attitude.

"When I approached their table, I put my one hand on my hip, and leaned back and pointed a finger right in the face of one of

9

the students that laughed. I said, 'Now look here you little punk, hear me out because there are some things I want to say, and I won't say it twice or stutter. First of all, let's make it perfectly clear: I'm not the one to take your shit! If you have a problem with me, we can deal with it right now, or back the hell off! You know, you need to act your age not your shoe size. Finally, don't let your mouth get my size-nine foot up your butt! You got it?'

"After I gave them a piece of my mind the students got quiet. Although I was pissed off, I finally had the time to think. I said to myself, 'Davanna, before you take this situation to the next level you better speak with an adult. You're in school and this situation could get real ugly.' So I left the cafeteria, went directly to the principal's office, and told her about all the disrespectful animal noises and jokes. I also told her that I got into one student's face.

"During the conversation I told the principal I had mixed feelings. At first I felt bad because students made fun of me. But then I got tired of being teased. Next, I copped attitude with one of the students and was ready to rip off his head and spit down his neck to shut him up for the rest of his life.

"I knew my thoughts were wrong, because in the back of my mind I could hear my nana. She'd always tell me, 'Remember, no matter what people say about you Davanna, you are a beautiful girl. Although we know you get mad, I want you to always act like a lady. Remember, beautiful is as beautiful does.'

"When I heard my nana's voice in my head, it made me stop in my tracks right when I was ready to rip that boy's head off. The principal apologized to me and said that kind of behavior was unacceptable. She gave me permission to eat lunch in the library for the rest of the school year. I thanked her because she understood what I was going through.

"I liked being able to eat my lunch and use the computer in the library at the same time. It was the perfect time to complete my homework assignments from my first, second, and third period classes. I really would have preferred to eat in the cafeteria. That way I could have met other students and made some friends. But it helped to talk to the principal. I felt very special, because someone really understood that I had real feelings."

"Cool," said Seth. "And give a high five to the principal who understood your feelings. That's great! Plus she took the time to support you. You know, I've had some broken feelings just like you did."

"Want to talk about it?" asked Davanna. She felt better after telling her friends everything.

"Okay," Seth answered. "I'm Seth Bernstein, a fifteen-year-old young man. Like Maritza, I'm in the tenth grade at Cedar Grove High. I live with my mom and my workaholic dad, outside of the city. We're Jewish and we go to a synagogue one day a week. I'm attractive, I'm smart, and I'm sarcastic. Oh! I forgot to mention that I'm somewhat round.

"Here's my question to y'all. Have you ever been treated like you were an invisible man? Or had people say bad things about you in your face, like you weren't even there?"

"Yes," Maritza replied. "I bet we all have." The others nodded.

"Well, I can remember a day when two attractive girls stood in front of me in the hall at school. As I walked toward them, one girl pointed her finger dead in my face and said, 'Ooh, you're cute.'

"As I began to feel happy about her compliment the other girl said, 'But I can't see the top of his pants, because his belt loops are trapped underneath that stomach.'

"Then they looked at each other and said, 'Yuck, he looks nasty.'"

Seth sat up and leaned closer towards his friends, talking faster now.

"There was another time when people looked me straight in the eyes and did not speak. I was standing in a whole group of people. When I spoke to people that I knew, they acted like I was invisible and hadn't said anything. But as soon as a skinny person came around, the same people made eye contact with them and held a full conversation. It was like I wasn't even there. I thought to myself, if those people took the time to know me they would know I'm a fun-loving person. The same way that y'all found out."

"C'mon now, Seth," said Maritza. "Who wouldn't want to talk to you, or be your friend? You know that you're all that and a bag of chips."

"That invisible thing has happened to me too," John added.

Seth continued. "If I had low self-esteem, I would've crawled under a rock and hid with the worms and frogs. But whenever I feel low, my mom says, 'Seth, there's no one in the world more important or talented as you. So do not let other people bring you down.' Her words keep me in check when people say ugly things to me. I believe every word of what she says."

Seth looked out at the waves crashing on the beach, and everyone thought about his story.

Then Maritza coughed. "So, Seth, you thought your story was bad, well let me tell you about mine. My name is Maritza Rodriquez. I am a fifteen-year-old Latina tenth grader at Cedar Grove High. I used to live in the suburbs, but moved into the city with my mom after my parents divorced. One thing that I am sure of is although I don't live with my dad, I still love him. When I visit him on weekends, they're happy visits. I believe I'm gorgeous, funny, and overweight. This is what happened to me.

"One day a friend and I walked to school. As we approached the school, two kids walking by us said, 'Hey you!'

"So we both turned around at the same time and asked, 'Who, me?' One kid said to my friend, 'Not you.'

"'Yeah, you!' the other kid yelled at me. 'The big one! You know Weebles wobble, but they never fall down.'

"Then they laughed until tears dropped from their eyes and snot was dripping from their noses. Do y'all know what Weebles are?"

"I don't," said John.

"They're egg-shaped toys that sit on a piece of curved metal. They don't have any arms and they're one big blob. No matter how hard you push them, they just roll from side to side. They won't fall down.

"After that, one of the kids said, 'You look like one of those girl Weebles.' And the other kid said, 'You're so round, I'll bet you can't fall down on that fat ass. You'll just bounce back up, just like a Weeble.'"

Maritza stopped talking for a minute and picked at the sand with her fingers. Then she looked up. "You know, I've been called a fat ass so much that I began to think that Fat Ass was my first name. I would ask myself, 'Why me, why me?' I used to be such a happy person, and I don't bother anyone.

"There was another day when I went into school and this guy said, 'Hey, big booty Judy! Do you know you got a big booty? I'll bet you when you stop walking that booty will still move. You know, there must be jelly back there in those jeans, because jam doesn't shake like that.'

14

"Then he laughed for a while. My first reaction was to turn around and say, 'Yeah, I might have a big booty, but I bet your mama has a big ole booty just like mine.' But I decided not to say it after all, because it was mean. And I didn't want to get into a fight.

"That guy wanted me to go back and forth with him and use negative words. But I realized that it wasn't worth it. What I should've done was report him to the principal for sexual harassment. Instead, I walked into the school and said nothing.

"I think my friend who was with me was more embarrassed for me than I was. When people like that guy tease me, I feel alone and get depressed. Most people don't take the time to see that I'm a kid just like them. I'm the same age, at the same school, doing the same things.

"Whenever I feel a little down, I hear Uncle Jose's voice in the back of my head. He says, 'Maritza, just ignore them. The kids who tease you have problems you can't see with your naked eyes. Their problems are deep inside. So baby, don't pay them any attention, and do not feel bad. Remember, be the best of whatever you are. And don't have any shame in your game.'

"When I think of his words, they put a smile on my face."

Maritza looked over at John. "You're the last one. You can start, because I'm finished with my story."

"Okay." John was ready. "My name is John Wong. I'm fourteen and in the ninth grade at Cedar Grove High. I'm Asian-

American and I live in the city with my down-to-earth dad. He's a single parent, because my mom died when I was ten. I'm a computer geek. I'm handsome, shy, and chunky. Just like you all, I have some tough stories because I'm heavy."

"Once I was in the restroom of a fancy restaurant. A kid came up to me and said, 'I can't understand why you are so damn fat. I thought the only thing y'all ate was rice. Man, if that rice you ate made you that damn fat, I'm going to tell the waitress to hold off on my rice!'

"That hurt for two reasons. First, the kid made fun of my weight. Then he stereotyped my culture when he said, 'All y'all ate was rice.' I was so mad I wanted to change from being a shy guy into a mean and evil guy. I really wanted to knock that kid's braces off his teeth. This was the first time I questioned myself about whether I needed to lose some pounds.

"When I used to go outside and play, kids would throw things at me and run. They would say, 'Ha ha, I bet you can't catch me. You're too fat to run.'

"Those kids made me real mad. But I remembered what my computer teacher, Mr. Abbott tells me. He says, 'Son, when someone does something to you that makes you feel bad, keep your head up. Walk tall with pride and never let them see you sweat!'

"It helps me to get past the worst feelings about being teased. Mr. Abbott also says, 'John, look at your life on the positive side. You do not have any physical or mental illness to slow you down. So when you look at a glass of water, you can see that glass as being halfway full, which is positive. Not half-empty, which is negative."

"I never realized that we were all being teased or bullied." Seth said.

The others nodded in agreement.

"Okay, now what should we do about it?" Maritza asked.

"I thought of talking to the school nurse," said Davanna. "But it's summertime so I can't even do that. But I have an idea! I'll call the clinic in my neighborhood. Maybe they have someone who could help us with being teased." She looked around at her friends. "But are we all ready to do something about it?"

One by one, each person nodded.

"So how do I describe us to the clinic?"

"Tell the clinic we're four teens who need to learn some strategies to use when people tease us," said Seth.

"That's great," Davanna answered. "And I just thought of a name for us. Let's call ourselves the We Can't Weight Teens. Because we're all so tired of being teased we can't wait til it stops. Do you get it, though? In We Can't Weight, its *weight* like heavy, not *wait* like waiting for a bus. What do y'all think about the name? Can we all agree to our new name?"

"Hum, I don't know. Does the word *weight* make sense? *Weight* like overweight," asked Maritza.

"Yes, it makes sense. We used it because of our size. Because that's why we're being teased."

"Oh, I got it," said Seth.

"Now I get it," Maritza said.

John added, "That's a cool way to say it."

"If we all agree, it's unanimous," said Davanna. We'll call ourselves the We Can't Weight Teens. Now, are we ready to get an appointment to discuss why we're being teased and what to do about it? I can go online and find the number for the neighborhood clinic."

"I think I can speak for all of us. We're ready," John whispered.

He didn't look like he was ready. Actually, he looked a little nervous. Everyone nodded. They would never feel totally ready. But they had to take a chance to see what happened. It was easier knowing they were all doing it together.

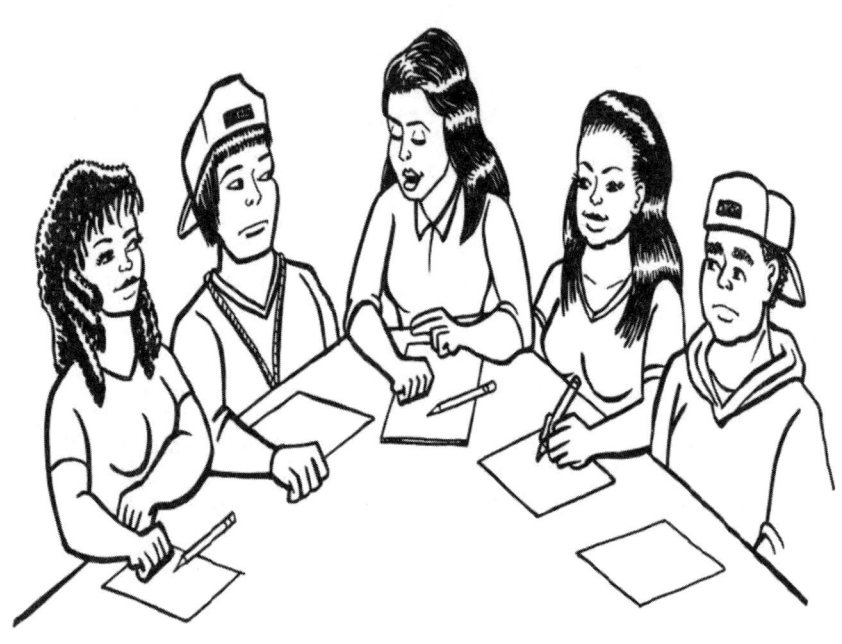

# CHAPTER THREE
## Why Were We Being Teased?

When Davanna called the neighborhood clinic, she told the receptionist about how the We Can't Weight Teens were being teased. The receptionist connected Davanna to a social worker named Ms. Lemon. On the phone Davanna described what was happening to her and her friends.

Ms. Lemon said very kindly, "Okay, I understand you. I would like to meet with the four of you. We'll talk for a while and figure out why you all are being teased. Then we'll agree on some strategies to be used in the future.

"I have an open appointment in my book for next Tuesday at nine a.m. Let's book the four of you in on that day. Check with your friends and call me if you need to find another time."

"Okay, Ms. Lemon, I think we'll be able to make it because this is important to all of us. Thank you for your support."

When Davanna hung up the phone, she felt like the world had been taken off of her shoulders. Ms. Lemon seemed to understand their problem and took it seriously. Davanna couldn't wait to tell her friends.

She went over to Seth's house where there was a three-way phone. They called Maritza and John, and Davanna told them all what had happened.

"Ms. Lemon's a social worker that called herself an MSW, go figure. So we have an appointment to meet with her at the clinic to talk about being teased. The appointment is next Tuesday. Can everyone make it?"

Everyone could be there. It was unanimous. They would meet with Ms. Lemon.

The week passed quickly, and on Tuesday, the We Can't Weight Teens went to the clinic. They were nervous as heck, but happy. They really hoped Ms. Lemon would help them find a way to stop being teased and disrespected.

After they sat in the waiting room area for a few minutes, Ms. Lemon came out to meet them. She seemed about seven feet tall! She had long wavy hair and pale fair skin.

"You must be the We Can't Weight Teens." Ms. Lemon spoke with a British accent. "Are you all ready for our meeting?"

The teens looked at each other, gulped, and nodded.

"Well, follow me."

As they followed her through a door and down a hall to her office, the four friends whispered to each other.

"Man, she's tall," said Davanna, looking her up and down. "We better not piss her off."

Maritza responded, "Yeah, she's a giant. She might just slam us."

"She could be a female basketball player," John said.

"I got it!" said Seth. She's as tall as the tree in my front yard."

"We can't be afraid of her. We have to remember the reason we're here," Davanna said firmly. "We need her help. Let's not think about how tall she is."

Ms. Lemon led them into a room with a long table and five chairs. She sat down with a lined notepad and pen in front of her. The We Can't Weight Teens sat at the table.

"Could we go around the table and have each of you tell me your name, your age, and a little something about you?"

"I guess I'll go first. My name is Davanna Brown and I am fourteen. I like to swim, play golf, and play guitar. Oh I forgot, I'm an A student who loves science, math, technology, and Justin Bieber. Can I add one more thing?"

"Yes you can," Ms. Lemon smiled.

"I live with my mom, dad, and brother outside of the city."

Ms. Lemon took notes and pointed to Maritza. "You're next, young lady."

"I'm Maritza and I'm fifteen. I love to watch baseball games, and my favorite singers are Beyoncé Knowles and Miley

Cyrus. I share my life with both of my parents. I live with my mom on the weekdays and my dad on the weekends."

Ms. Lemon wrote her notes and nodded at Seth.

"Hi Ms. Lemon, my name is Seth and I'm fifteen years old. I play baseball. I live with my workaholic dad and real cool mom in the suburbs about two miles outside the city."

"Okay, young man, you're the last one."

"Good morning, I'm John Wong and I am fourteen. I love to fix and work with computers. I've never come across one that I couldn't take apart and put back together. I also enjoy baseball. My dad and I moved into the city after my mom died."

"I'm sorry to hear about your mom," Ms. Lemon said.

"Thanks Ms. Lemon."

"Is there any more information you think I should know about? No? Then help me understand what's going on. How did the We Can't Weight Teens meet?"

"Well, we all go to a magnet school," explained Davanna. "It's open to students from different communities. So even though Seth and I live in the suburbs and Maritza and John live in the city, we met at school."

"You four must be good friends, if you spend time together during the summer."

"You can say that," Maritza said, smiling.

"Davanna called the clinic because you all were being teased. Is that right? When is that happening?"

"The real question should be when it is not happening," Seth replied.

"Yeah," John said. We get teased on a daily basis. Like when we walk to and from school, and in our neighborhoods, at restaurants, on the beach, or anytime we are in public. It doesn't stop."

"It just happened to us the other day at the beach," Seth added. "We were sitting there. We talked, laughed, and just had fun. Then a couple about our age walked by and called us a nasty name."

"What did they call you?"

John looked at Ms. Lemon like she was crazy. He couldn't believe that she, a social worker, was asking him to swear. "I'm sorry, but I can't repeat it to an adult."

"I'll repeat it," Davanna said. "We were lying on our beach towels. The couple walked by and said, 'Look at those fat asses.'"

Ms. Lemon looked at the others, who were surprised that Davanna actually said a swear word in front of an adult. "Is that what happened?"

"Yeah," they all said together.

"Then what did you all do?"

"Nothing," John, Maritza, and Seth said.

"But I did something!" said Davanna. "I was so mad that I jumped up and ran toward them and yelled, 'I got your fat asses alright!' Maritza, John, and Seth wrestled me down onto the sand.

24

That couple should consider themselves lucky that you three were there to hold me back."

"So Davanna, what were you going to do to the couple?" asked Ms. Lemon.

"I don't know, but whatever it was wouldn't have been nice."

"Are you telling me you would have hit one or both of them?"

Davanna said slowly, "It's possible."

Ms. Lemon looked at Davanna and rubbed her forehead with her hand. "Okay, Ms. Davanna. I don't want to have to send you to anger management classes for violent behavior. You need to start using other ways to deal with people when you are angry."

John asked, "But what should we do when we are being teased? I don't want Davanna to get into trouble because someone else disrespected her."

"Well, let's talk about some strategies you can be use instead of fighting. First, Davanna could have counted to ten and took deep breaths to calm down. When she reached ten, she might have had a little time to think about a different way to respond.

"Second, she could have chosen to walk away and ignore the couple. That's not always easy, and to use this strategy will require you all to do some deep soul-searching."

"Why?" asked Maritza.

"You need to understand that your problem is not with the people who tease you. Those people have personal problems hidden inside of them, just like you do. I don't blame you for having irrational thoughts when you are being teased, because it hurts. But the strategy to ignore the words and walk away allows you to stay out of trouble. Does that make sense?"

Everyone nodded.

"Let me ask a few more questions. I believe your answers will help me understand why that couple called you fat asses. Are you all ready?"

"I guess we are," said Davanna, looking at her friends. They nodded.

"What did the couple look like?"

"They were both tall and leggy," John responded.

"Were they attractive as you are?"

"The girl was cute. I don't remember the guy," Seth answered.

"What was their ethnic background?"

"They were Caucasian."

"Were they thick or thin?"

"They were undernourished. Skinny and bones like a skeleton," Davanna replied.

"Ah! I just figured out why the couple swore at you guys. Davanna just said both of them looked too skinny. Is that how all the We Can't Weight Teens viewed them?" Ms. Lemon asked, looking around.

Everyone nodded.

"And how do you think you four looked from the eyes of that thin couple?"

"I guess they thought we looked fat," Seth said slowly.

Ms. Lemon leaned back in her chair. "Seth just said why you all are being teased. It's that all of you are viewed by others as fat. Overweight. They make fun of you for it."

"But I'm not fat. I have thick bones," Maritza said.

"Everybody views weight differently," Ms. Lemon said. "But let's try something. We just have to go into the other room to do it."

The teens got up and followed Ms. Lemon. The next room had a scale, with a weight chart posted next to it.

Ms. Lemon pointed to the chart. "This is a weight chart. It shows the average normal weight each person should be based on their age and height. The average weight is determined by doctors and is based on science and health."

Ms. Lemon looked at each of the teens. "If you all allow me to measure your weight and then use the weight chart, I can determine whether you are overweight according to the average. Does anyone have a problem with me doing that?"

"No," everyone said.

Ms. Lemon weighed each person and measured the weight on the chart. Then she said, "Well, my guess was correct. You have something in common. According to the chart you are all overweight. But the good thing is that you're not obese."

"Go figure," Davanna whispered to Maritza, then asked, "Hey Ms. Lemon, how do you know we're overweight but not obese?"

"Well, for each age there's an average weight, which is the weight that it's healthiest to be. Above the average is overweight, when you're too heavy. Obese is above that, when you're way way too heavy."

Ms. Lemon walked to the cabinet against the wall and took out some pamphlets. "The clinic sent some information from the Center for Disease Control and Prevention, which is sometimes called the CDC. It provides the same set of steps I just used to determine if your weight was average, overweight, or obese. Do you mind if I read the information aloud to you?"

"Not at all. Go ahead," John replied.

"Please read it," said Davanna.

John and Maritza nodded.

"The pamphlet discusses how the body mass index, or BMI, value is charted for kids between the ages of two and nineteen. Each person has a BMI that is calculated using your weight, your age, and your height. That's what I figured out when I weighed each of you. Everyone has their own BMI."

She showed them the pamphlet. "The position of the dots here on the chart determines what percentile your BMI is in. The category of overweight is for people with a BMI that is at or above the eighty-fifth percentile but lower than the ninety-fifty percentile. The category of obese is for people with a BMI at or above the ninety-fifth percentile. Each one of you has a BMI that is lower than ninety-fifth percentile, but above the eighty-fifth. That's how I concluded that each of you was overweight not obese. Does that make sense?"

The four teens nodded their heads.

"So, I believe the issue for the We Can't Weight Teens issues is not about being teased or bullied. The real issue is that all of you are overweight. That's the reason people tease or bully you."

"But I don't want to be skin and bones like that girl on the beach," Maritza said.

"What do you think her BMI was?" asked Davanna.

Ms. Lemon thought. "Her BMI was probably somewhere between fourth and fifth percentile. If you all were to lose some weight, you wouldn't need to aim for that BMI. Just like it's possible to be overweight, it's also possible to be underweight, and that's not healthy either. I think you want to aim for a BMI between the fiftieth and eighty-fifth percentile.

"Also, I think you all have issues that connect to your being overweight. And if you tackle those issues, I believe you will stop being teased. What do you think?"

"Y'all, I think she's right," said John.

"Losing some weight is a part of that, but it's not the only thing," Ms. Lemon went on. "In order to tackle your overweight issues, you'll need to adopt some new mental and physical strategies. These strategies will forever change your lives and the way you look at food. Remember, I'm using the words 'overweight issues' and not 'overweight problem.' It's not just about losing weight. It's about deciding to change your old eating and exercise habits.

"Don't forget, your weight will not be lost overnight. Think about it, you didn't gain it overnight either. For some people, weight loss may be a slow process."

"Why?" asked Maritza.

"I like to say that weight loss is a 'you thing.' You have to want to lose the weight. Not because your mama, or daddy, or grandmother, or your friend wants you to. Your families can get rid of junk food and buy all the right foods and keep them at home. I'm talking about foods like sliced fruit and yogurt dip, celery slices and peanut butter, trail mix with raisins, nuts, and dried fruits. But if you're not ready to lose weight, you will continue to gain it. You might eat way more than you need to. And you might sneak and eat junk food, every chance you get, at school or at friends' houses or at restaurants.

"A lot of people continue their old habits and buy junk foods like soda, potato chips, cakes, cookies, and candy at the store on their way home. When they get home they eat it or hide it for later in a special place. Maybe you've seen the fire bear on TV? That bear says something like, 'Only you can prevent fires.' Well, Ms. Lemon's words are, 'Only you can decide to lose weight.'"

The four teens thought this over.

"Weight loss is a personal choice," Ms. Lemon continued. "Once you have chosen to lose the weight, you need to continue to adopt good eating habits. You also need to exercise daily. If you are committed to these two habits, the weight loss will happen. It begins with you making the choice. Do you want to make the choice?"

Davanna, Maritza, Seth, and John thought about it. They looked at the floor, they looked at the wall, and then they looked at each other.

"We're the We Can't Weight Teens," Davanna said. "Okay."

The others nodded. "Okay," they said.

"Great! I want to speak with Ms. Sussman from our nutrition department. Her knowledge and support has helped other teenagers adopt healthy eating habits and daily exercise regimens. I know teenagers who have followed her advice and brought their weight under control. The weight loss stopped them from being teased, and from hurting so badly. Trust me!"

Ms. Lemon walked to the door and then turned around and studied the four teens in front of her. "I'll go get Ms. Sussman now."

While she was gone, Davanna said, "I think we can change our eating habits and begin to exercise. But are we ready for this?"

"Yeah, I think we're ready," Maritza muttered. "But it kind of depends on what Ms. Sussman has to say."

Ms. Sussman walked into the room right then. She looked like she lifted weights. She was solid. There was not an ounce of fat on her entire six-foot-three chocolate body.

"Damn, are all of the staff members in this clinic giants?" Davanna whispered.

Ms. Sussman introduced herself and said, "I am the nutritionist here at the clinic. I heard you four are the We Can't Weight Teens. W-e-i-g-h-t. Is that correct?"

The teens nodded.

"I believe you guys knew you were overweight. That is why you adopted the name with *weight* spelled w-e-i-g-h-t instead of *wait*. Am I right?"

"That's possible," Davanna muttered.

"I think that's an interesting name. And I am glad you're ready to work on your weight issues. I'm going to give you some healthy ways to attack these issues." Ms. Sussman sat in her chair.

"But first let's go around the table and tell me your names so I know who you are."

The teens introduced themselves one by one.

"Thank you," Ms. Sussman said. "Now, I want to thank you all for being concerned about your weight." She rubbed her index finger across her chin and looked at them. "You all may not know it, but you are an attractive group. I am honored to put you on the path to losing weight. Before we begin, does anyone have questions? Don't be afraid to ask what's on your mind. There is no such thing as a dumb question. While I'm talking, if thoughts come to your mind, please feel free to interrupt me and share them with all of us."

"Do we have to go on a diet?" blurted out Davanna.

"Thank you, that's the number one question I get asked. The answer is no. Diets do not work. When people diet, they lose weight for a short period of time—the period of time they are on a diet. But, when that period is up and they stop the diet, the weight usually comes back. Remember, the purpose of a diet is to lose a few pounds over a short period of time. This is a quick fix, one that doesn't work for the rest of your life. Instead of a diet, it's better to make just two serious lifestyle changes."

Ms. Sussman had the teens' undivided attention.

"The first lifestyle change is to change your thoughts about unhealthy foods. Unhealthy foods are foods like fries, pizza, and soda. The second lifestyle change is to change how you eat and exercise. If you all agree to and focus on these two changes, you can lose weight."

No one spoke, but all four teens nodded their heads in agreement.

"Okay Ms. Sussman, those changes don't seem impossible. I think they can be done," Davanna said. "What are your thoughts, guys? Help a sister out."

"I think we could change our thoughts, and how we eat and exercise, if we did it over a period of time," said Seth. "You have to remember we didn't get these habits overnight."

"You're right Seth, we've had these habits for a long time. It's going to take some time to change," Maritza agreed.

"I agree with Davanna," said John. "The changes shouldn't be hard to do. Especially if it would stop us from being teased."

"Well Ms. Sussman, I think we all agree. The changes could be made over time." Davanna turned toward the nutritionist.

Ms. Sussman said, "Before you consider any new eating or exercising regimen you must check with your doctors. Each body is different, and your doctor will give you information that will support you when you are ready to make these lifestyle changes.

"Let me give you a few small suggestions. When you eat to lose weight, you must understand how to do it properly. Take your time. Chew your food slowly. Chewing slowly helps you eat less and taste your food. Instead of three big meals, try to eat six small meals. This will help you not to get hungry. Also, before each meal, drink a glass of water. That helps to fill you up and you won't want to eat as much.

"Also, remember that when you introduce your bodies to new foods you need to watch out for food allergies. If you eat foods that you are allergic to they can cause serious problems. Some of the foods that can sometimes cause allergic reactions contain gluten, peanuts, soy, eggs, milk products, or shellfish.

"I've worked with teenagers before and helped them lose weight. A few techniques helped them a lot. We talked earlier about changing the way you think about food.

"This new thought process will help you change your eating habits. The teens I worked with before now eat only when they're hungry, not just because food is there. Before, they ate three large meals. Now they eat six small meals that they prepare at home. Although the craving for junk food never goes away completely, they have learned how to substitute their cravings with healthy food. They snack on food from their six small meals as needed.

"Another thing they do is carry meals with them. They purchased soft lunch boxes and now they pack them at home so they can bring their food with them wherever they go. In the past they sometimes ate on the run. This eating habit forced them to choose unhealthy food, because they ate whatever was available to them at the time. After being taught to eat right, they fill their lunch boxes with cut-up apples, celery, carrot sticks, fruits, vegetables, and other healthy foods. Having these foods with them help prevent them from buying junk food. Each night before school, they put their snacks in plastic bags and keep them in the refrigerator until morning. The next morning, when they grab their homework and backpacks, they also grab their lunch boxes with snacks. When they get hungry or crave something to chew, they just have to reach into their lunch boxes to snack on healthy foods. On the days when they leave home without their snacks, they are tempted to buy junk food from the store or vending machines. Just like other teens, even though they know that junk food does not support weight loss.

"Another thing to remember is how important it is not to cheat or sneak unhealthy food."

"You mean not even one potato chip?" Davanna asked.

"No Davanna, chips are junk food," Maritza muttered.

"When those teens eat that one potato chip, the only one they really cheat is themselves. Each of you needs to keep that in mind. Because when those teens walk into their schools' cafeterias, they are strong and resist the temptation to eat junk food. They resist the vending machines and don't buy soda. Instead, they choose bottled water or drinks that contain 100 percent fruit juices. These are the healthy choices.

"To help you guys drink healthy liquids, play a little game with yourself. You could imagine that a bottled water or juice is actually a soda, or another beverage that you like to drink. When you drink it, it will quench your thirst but without as many calories as soda has.

"Also," Ms. Sussman continued, "It's important to remember that you shouldn't skip breakfast."

"What about a bagel on the run?" Seth asked.

"Nope. A bagel is not a complete breakfast. What you need to do is provide your body with enough needed nutrients, vitamins, and calcium. A bagel on the run is not the right balance. What you need from breakfast is to keep your body full until lunchtime.

"To do that, you should all pledge not to purchase caffeine drinks, soda, chips, donuts, or cinnamon rolls for breakfast. Instead, eat the school's breakfast. It provides healthier selections and it's free. But in order to eat breakfast at school, you must get there early, since it isn't served after nine in the morning. Here are a few examples of healthy breakfasts that can be made at home or are selections in school cafeterias. You can have one slice of raisin toast with one teaspoon of margarine. Sprinkle cinnamon on the top. Get a half-cup of sugar-free applesauce and a half-cup of milk. Or make a one-cup fruit smoothie out of fruits that you like, with a half-cup of dry cereal on the side."

"That means we couldn't meet outside of the school and talk to our friends," said Davanna. "That's where I hear all the gossip. We'd have to go into the cafeteria, sit down, and gossip as we ate."

"That's right, you will. And here's another important thing: the teens I've worked with before have changed from being inactive to getting physical exercise on a daily basis. They began with taking short walks, small weight routines, and swimming."

Davanna nodded her head and replied, "I can get with swimming."

"Hey Seth, you and I like to lift weights, so we can do that," Maritza responded.

"I like to walk," John added.

"That's great. Maybe you can find a few of your friends who would commit to walk with you. It helps to enjoy the company of your friends while you burn off calories. The best situation would be to have more than one committed friend, so you have at least one person ready to walk with you every day. If not, each one of you should learn to be your own best friend for exercise. Then you can swim, lift weights, or walk alone. Remember, you do not need a friend to help you burn off calories and lose weight. Weight loss is a 'you thing.'

"For walking, start off slow and work your way up to a brisk walk. Over time, you will get used to a long-distance walk. Your goal should be to walk for twenty to thirty minutes a day, either around the school track, on sidewalks, or in the park. Wherever you decide to walk, make sure it is in a safe area.

"If your family can afford to purchase a membership to a gym at the community center, YMCA or YWCA, the Boys and

Girls Club, or any other gym, you should do that. These places offer a lot of physical exercise classes that you can join. In order to lose weight, you must work out at least three times a week. Each session should be at least thirty minutes.

"If you like to swim, it's an excellent source of exercise. It forces you to use all of the muscles in your body. This is another way to burn off calories. Just like walking, with swimming you must start off slow. If you haven't been in the water for a while, you may get short of breath. So take your time. And remember that beginners must take swimming lessons to be safe. The important thing with swimming is not how fast you do it, but how long you are active in the water. Remember, your goal is to be active for twenty to thirty minutes. We have an awesome pool in our community center down the street, and I can help you get access to it as well as the gymnasium there. All you have to do is be ready to use them.

"I'll help you," Ms. Sussman told the four friends. "We'll work together."

Over the next several weeks, the We Can't Weight Teens had a lot of discussions with Ms. Sussman. One day they decided to meet at John's house to brainstorm about how they were going to lose weight.

"Can y'all believe that the first time we went to the clinic we went to talk about being teased?" asked Davanna. "Only to find out that being overweight was the real issue. That's some stuff.

Now that we know weight is our issue, and after all the things that Ms. Sussman told us about how to lose it, we know what we need to do. Here are my thoughts on how to do it. We should pick one day a week to meet and brainstorm about our weight goals. When we've agreed on the goals, we can find ways to achieve them."

"We can write everything down," said Seth.

"Yes, we'll write the goals on a big piece of paper and put it on the wall, like the one we had in our English classes."

"That way we can always see them," Maritza added.

"If we write them, it'll remind us of the time and energy it took for us to brainstorm about them," Davanna added. "Also, if we see them all the time, we won't be able to forget them. It will help us stay motivated to do what we wrote down."

"The other day I was online, and I went to the President's Challenge website. It had something called an active lifestyle activity log. We can download it to write down our weekly activities."

"What was the website?" John asked.

She wrote it down for him. It was www.presidentschallenge.org.

"What do we do once we've made the log?" asked Seth.

"Then we physically use our goals to lose weight. I mean physically, for real. Let's pick a day, like Monday, that's a good day to meet, and meet each week to plan our exercise. We can meet at a different person's house and each time that person can make sure to have healthy snacks there for us to eat. Okay? Can we agree to meet Mondays?" Davanna asked.

"I guess so," Seth said.

"What about you two, Maritza and John? Mondays?" Maritza nodded her head.

"Okay Davanna, we'll do it," John said.

"The summer will be over and we'll be back in school. We'll have to pick a time that gives us enough time to finish homework. Could y'all raise your hand to vote on the time that's best to meet? Three-thirty? Four? Four-thirty?"

They all raised their hand for four-o'clock, because it allowed them enough time to get their homework done before the meetings.

"Alright, those were my suggestions," Davanna said. "Now everyone else should give theirs."

"Maybe we can meet three times a week and walk around the track!" Seth said. "Each time we can walk for twenty to thirty minutes. Ms. Sussman said that was a good way to burn off calories."

"Great!" said Davanna. "So we'll meet more days each week. We're already meeting on Mondays. Will Tuesday, Wednesday, and Thursday be too much?"

"I don't know about you all, but that's four days a week," Maritza muttered. "After going to school all day and doing homework, that's a lot."

"Okay, let's vote. Who wants to meet four days a week?"

Everyone raised their hands except Maritza.

"Davanna, I still think that's a lot of days," Maritza moaned.

"C'mon, we'll have the rest of the week and weekends to ourselves," John said.

"Yeah we will!" Davanna yelled. "But remember, the days we don't meet doesn't mean that we stop at our weight goals and just sit on our butts. We still have to work on our goals on Fridays, Saturdays, and Sundays. Does anyone disagree?"

The three others shrugged their shoulders. But no one disagreed.

Maritza whispered in Seth's ear, "Davanna's a little too serious about this weight thing. The next thing you know, she'll want us to meet on Fridays and Saturdays too."

Seth whispered back, "Yeah, she's very serious. If we want to stop being teased and bullied, we should be serious too."

Davanna was saying, "Since nobody disagreed, our plan is to meet on Mondays, Tuesdays, Wednesdays, and Thursdays to deal with our weight issues. And we need to continue working on our weight goals every day of the week, even when we don't meet. Does anyone else have another suggestion?"

John whispered to Maritza and Seth, "Hell no, I don't have any more suggestions. And you two better not give her any more ideas either."

"How about we write down everything we eat each day and bring it to our Monday meetings, so we can see how each person is doing?" Maritza asked.

"Great, Maritza! I saw a food record on the Internet. It had a blank form we could download and use." She wrote down the website and passed it around. It was http://facultyfiles.deanza.edu/gems/milleranna/Blankform.doc.

"Hey Maritza, I thought we weren't going to give her any more suggestions," Seth said.

Davanna didn't hear him. "How about you John, what's your suggestion?"

John rubbed his chin with his thumb. After some thought he said, "What if we weigh ourselves at our Monday meetings? That way we can find out if we gained or lost weight."

"Are you serious, weigh ourselves? In front of everyone?"

"Yeah, Maritza, what's wrong with that?"

"Now that's too personal," she mumbled.

"C'mon Maritza, it's going to be okay," John responded. "This is between us."

"Look y'all, how else would we know if our weekly meetings are working?"

Everyone looked at Davanna and rolled their eyes. But they knew she was right. What other measurement could they use to determine if they had lost weight?

"Oh, what the heck, we'll weigh ourselves on Mondays," Maritza said.

"It would be a good idea if we each brought a notebook to write down our true weights. Then we can write down our goal weights and anything else we want to share with the group."

"Okay," everyone said.

"I have another question," Davanna said.

"Oh, no, here she goes again," Seth said.

"Had any of us ever told our story to anyone?" Davanna asked. "The story of how we became overweight?"

"I don't think so," answered Maritza slowly. "Not exactly."

"Nope," Seth moaned, worried about what Davanna was getting at.

"I know I never told a soul," said Davanna. "Y'all know what I think?"

"I can't even imagine," Maritza sighed.

"Well, I think it's about time for us to dig deep into our souls and tell our stories."

"What stories again?" asked John.

"The stories of our issues. John, we could tell the world the reasons why we became overweight. Just think about it. There may be other teens that had the same experiences we did. They need to know they're not alone, and shouldn't be ashamed of what's happened to them. You know what?"

"No, I don't. But I bet you're going to tell us," said Maritza. "What great idea do you have up your sleeve now?"

"The point is that our stories may help other people understand they're not the only ones who've experienced major drama in their lives. Don't you agree?"

"I never thought about it like that," Seth agreed.

The room was silent.

"It's been a lonely journey so far," said John finally.

"You're so right. There must be people who are hurting in silence, just like I was," Maritza whispered. "I think it's time for me to tell my story. I'm with you, Davanna."

"Okay. Since we all agree, it's time to get started. We'll each tell our stories. We'll shout them out!" Davanna yelled. "If y'all don't mind, I'll go first."

# CHAPTER FOUR

## Our Reasons for Being Overweight

*Davanna's Story*

Some people thought I was thick or fat because I loved to eat. Don't even believe it! There were other reasons for me being overweight and I'm going to share them with you. I can think of two big reasons that I started to eat all of the time and became overweight.

The first began when my mom and dad moved from where I was born to another state. This move caused major problems for me. I used to spend a lot of time with my dad's family, like my nana and my auntie. We were so close. When I was born they were all in the delivery room. They helped my mom push me out of her body!

But one day Mom and Dad decided to move us to another state. They didn't tell me, or Nana, or Auntie. I was young, but I still remember it. I was supposed to visit Nana's house that weekend. I saw her every week. I was all hyped up, because I was going to see her. She and Auntie used to spoil me.

As I packed my bag, my mom said, "Davanna, you're not going to Nana's this weekend, because we are moving."

For me, moving was not a problem. We'd moved on a regular basis. I thought the move wouldn't be too far from my nana's house. But then Mom broke the bad news.

"We are moving far away and you'll have to catch an airplane to see Nana and Auntie."

"An airplane!" I yelled, "Did you tell Nana?"

"No."

"What do you mean *no*?"

That's when my whole world crumbled, when my parents took me away from the rest of my family. What was even worse, they didn't even tell Nana and Auntie about the move until after we moved. So I didn't get to say goodbye. Believe me, that sucked.

I was really close to my dad's side of the family. Every time I thought of them, I missed them. I fell apart. I cried. I felt lonely, upset, and depressed because I missed them so much.

It got so with each thought of missing them, I ate. I didn't eat because I was hungry, I ate because I felt like I had a hole inside of me, and the only thing that filled this hole was food. The more I ate the bigger I got. Food became my best friend for when I missed my family.

After we moved, I used to visit Nana and Auntie. I saw them on Thanksgiving, Christmas, and some of my summer vacations. But three times a year was not enough. I always felt so special on my visits that I didn't want to go back home to my mom and dad. Nana and Auntie treated me like a princess. But when I was away from my parents for a long time, I missed them too. So it was hard both ways.

The second reason I became overweight was that I love fast food. I get busy when I eat a double cheeseburger and fries. And eating fast food became a habit. Each day on the way home from school, I stopped at one of my favorite fast-food restaurants and ordered a double cheeseburger, fries, a milk shake, and dessert. I left the restaurant as soon as they gave me my food, because cold fries taste horrible. And warming them in the microwave makes them taste the worst! So, as soon as I got home with my hot food, I ate it fast while I worked on my homework. When I finished homework, I turned on the computer until suppertime.

Each night my family sat down and ate supper. Then I played video games, and just before bed I watched TV. All of that means that I sat on my big butt from the time I came in from school all the way until bedtime. Beside me would be junk food that I bought on the way home. My parents didn't buy junk food, but I did. Every chance I got, I would sneak and eat some. I got heavier and lazier.

My mom and dad were different. They were active as hell, and in great shape. They went to the gym three times a week and walked each day. They tried to enroll me in a gym for teens and take me for daily walks with them. When they asked me, I always made up an excuse explaining why I couldn't go. I said I had to do homework or told them I had menstrual cramps.

Sometimes I looked at them and asked myself, Why me, why me? Why do I have to be so big when they're so slim?

Then reality sunk in. They were physically active and I was not. Duh! For many years my parents tried to help me lose weight. They would buy skim milk, low-fat ice cream, fifty-percent-reduced-fat salted pretzels, all natural applesauce, and air-popped popcorn, because it's high in fiber and low in calories.

Also, they made all our desserts themselves, so my mom controlled the amount of sugar in each recipe. At home I ate healthy. But when I could, I bought all the junk food I could find, because I liked how it tasted.

To help me lose weight, my mom and I went to a weight-loss program that my doctor recommended. Together my doctor and my parents told me about the medical issues that come from being overweight. These are diseases like diabetes, sleep apnea, high blood pressure, and damaged arteries. We also talked about physical problems like shortness of breath, which was starting to happen when I walked, played in the gym, or when I was trying to sleep.

My parents were also concerned about the social challenges that come with being overweight. Like me being insecure about how I looked. My size didn't allow me to wear stylish clothes. My parents asked me who would I date, since a lot of people like thin girls. Would I date anyone who told me I was cute, they wondered? Would I fall in love with a playa, just because he told me he loved me? They worried that for an overweight teen, the selection of guys or girls would not be great. Their greatest fear was that I would date someone and not take the time to get to know him or her. And not knowing someone could lead to major problems like date rape or physical or emotional abuse. So, they were scared.

They continued to talk to me about overweight teens who had abused drugs and alcohol just to fit in with the more popular crowd. These were some of the same teens who had thoughts of suicide. You'd think, with all of that information, that I could have gotten it together. Nope, I didn't.

One thing I began to realize when we started talking to Ms. Sussman was that all of my parent's advice meant nothing to me until I was ready to lose the weight. I'm fourteen, five feet three inches tall, and weigh a hundred and thirty-five pounds. My BMI is twenty-three, which is in the eighty-seventh percentile. So that puts me in the overweight not obese category. And that means that eighty-seven percent of teenagers who are my age, weight, and height have BMI numbers lower than mine.

Snap, that's scary. I began imagining that if there were eighty-seven teens standing around me, all of them would have a BMI below mine. Damn. So I said to me, "Self, you've got to do something about your weight, because this is crazy."

I believe I'm ready to stop sneak eating. The burgers and fries that I used to eat? I'm going to leave them alone. Now is the time to conquer my weight issues.

## Seth's Story

I lived with my mom and dad, in what I believed to be a normal family. Although Mom had a part-time job, she made sure she was always home when I left for school and home when I got back from school. She planned her hours at work to be from eight to two because she didn't want me to be home alone or become a latchkey kid.

She would always say, "When kids are home alone, they get into trouble." She wanted to protect me and hoped that I would do the right thing when she was not around.

My afternoon routine was to come home, shut off my cell phone, and wash my face and hands. Then I grabbed the snack my mom always had prepared for me and went to the study to complete my homework. While I did that, mom prepared dinner and a dessert. The food smelled so good, sometimes it interfered with my thoughts. Yes, she cooked her butt off, and my size showed it. From what you just heard, you could tell that Mom and I had a great relationship. However, the relationship with my dad was the total opposite.

Each day about five-thirty, Dad came in from work. He barely spoke to Mom and me. We'd say hi, and he would just grunt, "Yeah!"

Dad was like a robot. He grunted at us, washed his hands, grabbed his newspaper, and sat down at the table for dinner. While we ate he focused on the paper and never looked up at us. He always finished the paper and dinner at the same time. When he was done, he wiped his mouth with a napkin, went into the family room, and sat in front of the TV until he fell asleep.

If I asked him a question, he'd say, "Leave me alone. I'm tired." If my mom asked him a question, he would just grunt.

Each night Mom woke him up and made him go upstairs to take a shower and go to bed. He never talked to me, did anything with me, or took me anywhere. All he ever said was, "Leave me alone."

When he said that, it would hurt my feelings. He was my dad! I felt so bad that sometimes I went upstairs to my room and cried. Sometimes after a long cry, I'd go back to the kitchen and eat a lot of food. Like leftovers from supper, or cake, or cookies, or anything in the kitchen I could get my hands on. I even ate food I didn't like. Sometimes, I thought my dad didn't love me and that his heart was as cold as ice. I don't know why Mom kept him around, because he treated me like dirt or something that he just stepped on.

He never physically abused me or my mom, and he never said mean things about us. But there were many times he acted like we were invisible. He only talked to us if he were around when we were speaking with other people. Those times, he would interrupt the conversation and he always acted like he was the expert on the topic.

Each time I thought about how he treated me, I felt bad inside. So, I just ate. On weekends when you might think he would spend some time with Mom and me, he left the house before we got up and stayed out with his friends from morning to night. If Mom called him, he came home. However, if she never called him, he would stay out from Friday after work until Sunday night. When he finally came home, he smelled like alcohol. He tried to hide the smell by chewing gum or breath mints. Mom knew he drank, but always asked him, "Have you been drinking?"

And he always answered, "No. Why do you always ask me that question? It's like you don't believe me."

"If you didn't come in the house smelling like the liquor store, I wouldn't."

Dad always denied that he drank. One evening he asked me to get his slippers from his closet. As I looked through the closet, I found a bottle of liquor in the back. It was stashed away in one of his suit pockets. When I asked him about it he said, "Boy, you must be crazy. You did not find a bottle of liquor in my suit pocket. Stop playing before your mother believes you."

Then he went upstairs to his closet. He must have removed the bottle, because he called me up there. "Seth, come up here, boy."

When were both in front of his closet he said, "Now show me the suit with the bottle of liquor in it. Show it to me now."

Of course, the bottle wasn't there. He'd taken it out before I got there. He made it seem like I lied. I told mom about it.

She said, "Seth, you do not have to prove anything. I believe you. Your dad has had a drinking problem for quite some time, and he needed to get help long ago."

I thought about what she told me all night. The next day, I decided to talk to my dad about the Alcoholics Anonymous program. It's called AA and it's for people who have drinking problems. But before I got up the courage to talk to him, I looked at my dad and sized him up. Then I looked at me in the mirror. I thought to myself, "You know, Dad's kind of thin and I'm thick-boned. He's old and I'm fifteen. I'm five feet five, a hundred and fifty pounds, with a BMI of twenty-five. I'm overweight, what do I have to worry about?" Although he had never hit me, I believed I could hold him down with my weight if I had to.

It was Monday night and Dad came into the house and began his normal routine. Mom and I said good evening to him. Dad did his usual grunt, washed his hands, grabbed the newspaper, and sat down at the table for supper.

Before he began reading I said, "Hey Dad, I have to talk to you about something."

"Yeah, what's up?"

"Dad, for the last two or three years you go out and come home smelling like you've been drinking."

"Now that's none of your business, son. When you get old enough to work, buy a house, and pay your own bills, you too can have a drink or two. Don't forget, I'm the dad and you're the son. Get it?"

"You're right, Dad, but as your son, it is my business. I would like to talk to you about the AA program."

When he turned and looked at me he gave the evil eye. I thought he was going to yell until his brain exploded. But instead, he grumbled. "Yeah, I heard about AA."

The pamphlet I had gotten from my guidance counselor at school said that AA is a free program that helps people who drink get better. The goal of AA is to discuss the reasons why people drink and give them support or guidance to help them stop. I looked on the Internet and found an AA program in our community. There was a meeting at the community center down the street.

I told all this to my dad and said, "I wouldn't have a problem going with you to the meetings. Especially if it would help you deal with your drinking problem. Mom and I know you drink. That's why you leave the house early on the weekends and hang out with your friends. You meet them and drink. They're your drinking buddies.

"One day," I said to my dad, "I followed you to the spot where y'all hung out. When you arrived, all of your buddies were already drunk. So if you hang with them, you're drinking too. Remember you told me you're known by the company you keep? Well, the company you keep on weekends is drunk. Therefore, you must be a drunk too."

My dad looked at me carefully. He said, "I could get mad at you and tell you to shut up and mind your own business. But you're right, this is your business. I haven't known how to tell your mother or you that it's hard for me not to drink. I think I'm an alcoholic. I have been one for the past two or three years. I've tried to hide it by not talking to you when I'm at home. I know you both thought I didn't love and care about you, but I do. I just haven't shown it."

It had been so many years since I'd waited for him to say those words. It felt so good. I told my dad I loved him too. I asked him why he drank.

"You see, I had a lot on my mind. But even though that's true, it's not an excuse to get drunk. Being drunk did not fix my problems. In fact, it made many problems worse. But the liquor temporarily relaxed me, and kept me at a distance from negative thoughts. Son, did you think I was an alcoholic?"

"Yes, I did."

"I'm proud of you for being so direct. You stepped up to the plate and told me about my drinking problem. It took courage to go up to your ole man and say that."

"Yes, it did." I relaxed a little bit. "It took a whole lot of courage." I didn't tell him that I had already sized him up, in case he got physical.

"Seth, later this week we'll go together to the community center and see if I can get help with my drinking problem. I wasted a lot of time that I could have spent with you and your mother. Trust me, the wasted time will be made up to both of you. I also spent a lot of money on liquor. The money I spent on that could have paid off many of my bills."

"So Dad, if you believe in what you just said, let's go get this problem under control."

"I'm with you."

After he attended several AA meetings, my dad told me how much he loved me. We began to spend a lot of time together. But you know what? If y'all think someone you love is an alcoholic, my suggestion is don't be afraid to talk to them about it. Your conversation and support could be what is needed for the person to understand that they need help.

It seemed like my dad had been waiting for someone to say something to him about his drinking. When I spoke to my dad about it, it helped him be ready to attack his problem. Now, he and I spend time together. Go figure, now that we are together, he doesn't go out with his friends on the weekends. When he gave up drinking, I knew it was time for me to give up eating. So, it's time for me to knock off these pounds.

*Maritza's Story*

Mom, Dad, and I used to live in our beautiful home in the suburbs. We had the white picket fence and all. We were a happy family, so I thought.

One day, my parents sat me down and told me that they were going to get a divorce, because they did not get along like they used to. I was shocked, since they never argued or said mean things to each other. After that conversation, I began to notice different things. Dad came home from work, changed his clothes, and went out for the night. Mom stopped setting a plate for him. One morning as I ate breakfast I saw a letter on the table. The letter was from family court. So I read it. There was a date and time for us to go to court. I was included in the "us."

The court was a huge concrete building with a lot of offices and back-to-back courtrooms. The ceilings had big gargoyles that sat up there and glared down at me. It was a scary place. It looked like a building in a sci-fi movie. An officer took us into this small courtroom. There was a male judge dressed in a black dress. At first I thought the judge was crazy because the only other time I had ever seen a man in a dress or skirt was watching the Scottish bagpipers on TV. They wear pleated skirts that they call kilts.

I'd never been inside of a courtroom. It was all new to me. I met two people there. One was a lady, who was my mom's lawyer. The other was a man, my dad's lawyer. The lawyers talked to each other. Then they went up to the judge's bench. The judge whispered some words to both lawyers. I guess he didn't want Mom, Dad, and me to hear what they planned for my family. Then the lawyers came back and talked to my parents. After Dad's lawyer talked to him, I noticed a tear dropped from his eye. But I didn't understand why. When it was over, Mom said, "Maritza, give Dad a kiss goodbye."

I thought, "What the heck just happened? We all came into the court together. There wasn't a fight. Kiss him goodbye? Did Dad's lawyer tell him to leave town? Was he going to jail? What the heck?"

"The judge wants Dad and me to be separated from each other before the divorce," Mom said. "So, you will move with me into an apartment in the city. Dad's going to live in another house."

"What! That judge said all of that?"

"That was what he told the two lawyers."

I was devastated and angry. "Mom," I said, "I should go up to that judge and give him a piece of my mind. Tell him to mind his own business, because he doesn't even know my family. Why didn't he ask to speak to me? Oh, I guess because I'm a teenager, and how I feel doesn't matter. Go figure. Am I going to see Dad anymore?"

"Yes, of course. But only on the weekends."

"So you're telling me I have to have a part-time dad?"

"No. He'll still be your dad all of the time. You can call him whenever you want to."

I felt really bad. I'm a daddy's girl who used to wait each night for him to come home from work. He was a part of my daily routine. Every day I would come home from school, do my homework, and watch a little TV. Then I would wait for the six o'clock news to end. Not that I liked the news, but when it was over, Dad came through the door and held me in his arms.

Don't misunderstand, I loved my mom too. But my dad was the best. Now that he wouldn't live with us everything would be different.

After I lived with just my mom, I would daydream about my dad. As I daydreamed, I ate anything and everything that was in sight. I ate even though I was not hungry. I ate every time I missed my dad. That was a lot. My mom and dad noticed that I was depressed and was overeating. They knew I was having a hard time dealing with their legal separation. Although they were separated, they did not rush to file for a divorce. Instead, they thought we should all go to a family counselor. Their goal was to solve their problems, so one day we could become a family again, which would be better for all of us. But, they knew everything would take time.

There's another reason I became overweight, and it was horrible. After mom and I moved to the city she met this guy and they started to date. He was always nice to me and gave me anything I wanted. Sort of like my dad. He dated Mom for a year, so we both got to be comfortable with him. The three of us talked, played board games, and watched TV together.

One Thursday, Mom was out at an appointment at the clinic. When I got home, she wasn't there, but her boyfriend was. He told me, "Your mom will be back in about an hour and I'll watch you until then."

That was cool. As usual, I got a snack and began my homework. When I finished, I went into the family room and watched TV. Mom's boyfriend came in and sat down next to me. That was normal, that happened all the time. What was not normal was what happened next. While we watched TV, he moved closer and closer to me. He took one of his arms and put it around my shoulder.

I looked at him like he was crazy. So he took his arm away. But then he rubbed my right arm up and down with his hand. At first I thought, "This man must be crazy." Then I thought, "Oh hell no, this man is some kind of freak." That made me nervous. I was very concerned.

After he rubbed my arm for a while, he slid his hand down onto my jeans. Then he touched my private area. By this time I was more than nervous, I was uncomfortable and confused. He had been in my house many times before, but he never did anything like that.

Then I realized this was the first time I was alone with him. Before that, my mom had always been there too.

He took his hand and put it inside of my jeans underneath my underwear. I was so scared that I froze. I screamed, but no sounds came out of my mouth.

At the time I was just twelve years old. I believe I was five-foot three and weighed about one hundred fifteen pounds. Even though I gained some weight after my dad moved, I was still a thin little girl. I didn't think I could fight that guy off even if I could unfreeze long enough to do it.

Now it's three years later and I'm fifteen, five-foot four, and a hundred and forty pounds. My BMI is twenty-four. Yes, I'm an overweight young lady. With these extra twenty-five pounds, I could have kicked that guy's butt. But I don't think I could have given him the beat-down that he really needed. He needed his butt kicked by someone his own size.

During the time he touched me, I thought, "This is terrible. I'm being touched in my private area, in my own house! And neither my mom nor my dad is here to save me."

Finally, he took his hand away and squeezed my face with his other hand and said, "Listen to me, this is our little secret. You better not tell anyone. If you do, I'll hurt your mom, you got it?"

I said yes. I was ashamed, embarrassed, and humiliated. And I was scared. I thought it was my fault that he did that mean thing to me.

I asked myself, "Did I wear the wrong clothes? Were my jeans too tight? Was it my mom's perfume that I snuck and sprayed on me without her permission?" I didn't and still don't understand.

I also blamed my mom because she left me alone at home with him. And I blamed my dad, because he no longer lived with us. He didn't walk through the door as he used to, right after the six o'clock news. If he had he could have saved me from the freak. Each time I thought of that horrible time, I ate like I never ate before.

I told my mom what happened when she got home that night. I said, "Mom your boyfriend put his hand into my pants and underwear."

"Maritza, why are you lying on that man?"

"I'm not lying, Mom! He really did. It happened while we watched TV."

Guess what, she didn't believe me. I could not believe that my own mom didn't believe her only daughter. She called me a liar! I felt real bad. I thought no one would ever believe me. But the next day was Friday and I was going to my dad's house. I knew he would believe me, but I was scared to tell him.

As usual, Dad picked me up from school. When I saw him I ran to him as fast as I could. I jumped into his arms. He kissed me and I hugged his neck. But when I did not let go of his neck, he asked, "Maritza, are you okay?"

At first I didn't say anything, but started crying. Dad noticed a change in me. He put me down and knelt down so that we looked at each other face to face.

"Maritza, look me in the eye and tell what's wrong."

"Okay. Mom's boyfriend put his hand into my underwear."

"What did you say? He did what?"

"He put his hand in my underwear."

Dad put his hand on his forehead and walked back and forth up and down the sidewalk. Then he asked me, "Did you tell your mother?"

"Yes, I did. But she didn't believe me."

He opened his eyes until his eyebrows went into his hairline. Then he continued to walk up and down the sidewalk. "What do you mean, she didn't believe you?"

"When I told her what he did, she didn't believe me."

Dad put his hands on my shoulders. "I want you to understand me, baby. Daddy believes you."

"I had on my skinny jeans and they were really tight. Maybe I shouldn't have been wearing them."

"There was nothing wrong with your jeans or anything else you could have worn. There is no way this was your fault, okay? That's a grown man who has touched my daughter. Do you know how to get to his house?"

"No, I don't."

As I looked into Dad's eyes, it looked like the white part of his eyes had turned blood red. He was so mad I got scared.

He repeated, "Maritza, I want you to know that what happened to you was not your fault. Never let anyone tell you that it was. Is that understood?"

"Yes Dad, it's understood."

"But don't you worry. Daddy will take care of this problem."

Dad drove me to the police station and told the police lady there what Mom's boyfriend had done. The police lady asked me a lot of questions and said, "Maritza, you did not do anything wrong. When we find him, you can be sure that he will not ever do that to you or anyone else again."

I didn't really know what she meant, but I believed her. While we were in the police station, Dad called my mom. They talked for a good while.

I heard Dad ask Mom, "Do you know what your boyfriend did to our daughter? Huh! Do you know? Okay, okay, I don't want to hear any reasons. Where does he live? Just tell me, where does he live?"

Finally, Mom told Dad her boyfriend's address. The police lady put her hand on Dad's shoulder and told him, "Mr. Rodriguez, do not do anything to that man. Please do not take the law into your own hands. Let us take care of him."

"But that's my daughter."

"I know that. Let me do my job."

"I'll try, but I cannot promise you," Dad said. He was really mad. "I hope you get to him before I do."

The police went to Mom's boyfriend's house and arrested him for what he did to me. Mom met us at the police station before they brought him back. After she arrived, two police came in with her boyfriend in handcuffs and asked me, "Is this the man who touched you in your private area?"

"Yes, that's him."

When I said that, my dad dashed toward him.

Dad said, "You nasty son of a bitch, you touched my daughter! You touched my baby!"

The two police grabbed my dad and held him against the wall. They said, "Mr. Rodriguez, we have him. We have him now. Just let us do our job."

Before the police grabbed Dad, I thought he was going to break the law. I felt his anger. As the police led the freak out of the room to go to jail, he gave me a mean look. He knew that I told his little secret. But I felt a lot safer, because I knew that he wouldn't ever touch me or another young lady.

When we left the police station, my parents took me to the hospital to get a checkup. The hospital told my parents I would be fine and made an appointment for me to talk with a counselor in the clinic.

All of that drama was so horrible. But after we left the hospital, Dad came over to our apartment. When he came inside he looked around and said, "You ladies don't have to worry about him anymore. My next move will be right here. I left before, but I will never leave you two again. Maritza, my baby, I'm so sorry for what happened. I should have been here to protect you and I wasn't. Please forgive me."

"I already forgave you, Dad," I said.

After my dad apologized, Mom felt really bad because she didn't believe me. She broke down into tears. She said, "Maritza, I'm so sorry that I didn't believe you. It's not your fault. I just didn't want to be alone. I was used to having your dad around. When we separated, I was lonely. That's why I didn't want to believe that my boyfriend would do something so horrible to you. Please forgive me."

At that time, I could not forgive her. But now I can. And with my dad home, I'm not afraid. Still, when I think about that freak and what he did to me, sometimes I feel so bad. For a long time, I thought eating would make me feel better, like it did when dad moved out. So I ate a lot.

A lot of boys and girls get touched in their private areas inappropriately. And it often comes from someone they know and trusted. A lot of times it's a family member or a friend. If the kid doesn't tell, the adult gets away with this terrible act. That means the adult can move on to the next child or teenager and do the same thing. Mom's boyfriend got arrested because I told the "little secret" that he told me to keep. He threatened to hurt my mom if I told! But he did that to make me scared. It was hard to tell, but it would have been worse if I never said anything.

I learned that it's okay to tell an adult if somebody touches you where he or she is not supposed to. If I couldn't tell someone in my family, I could have told a doctor, teacher, principal, or an adult in my school. These are the people who can help. It's their job to help if someone comes to them and tells them that.

This couldn't be a better time for me to tackle my weight issue, because I know that eating too much food doesn't make me feel better about myself. It makes me feel worse. I'm ready to get back to feeling good about myself.


*John's Story*

Let me tell you how it used to be. I used to be tall, fine, and thin. Sort of like Shaggy on the Scooby-Doo cartoons. The girls loved me. They chased me around and asked, "What's your name? Can I have your phone number? Hey, do you know how fine you are? Do you have a girlfriend?"

That was my life. It was wonderful. Things were great! But then my wonderful life took a major turn for the worse. It was my mom. She got diagnosed with cancer.

Now, you know guys have strong feelings for their moms. My mom made me feel important. My whole family depended on her to keep things running. She made us so happy.

Have you ever noticed how a person gets upset if someone talks about his mom? All hell breaks loose. Like when someone tells a nasty joke and then says, "Your mama." The first reaction is, "Oh hell no, I know you didn't just say that about my mama."

Well, that's how it used to be for me with my mom. I'm a quiet type of guy, but if someone talked about my mom I got crazy. She was that sacred person who was off-limits to disrespect or make jokes about.

Mom, Dad, and I used to sit down at the table for breakfast and dinner. We'd catch up on what had happened in each other's lives. We had happy family times. When Mom got cancer, our family times were shattered like broken glass. If you've ever accidentally broken someone's window or dropped a mirror, maybe you remember how the glass shattered. You can see the shape of it, the center of the shattered part where the glass was hit or dropped, radiating out to the edges.

All you could do if the glass breaks is put your hand over your mouth, raise your eyebrows, and say, "I'm in big trouble." It was scary because you knew the trouble had consequences.

As quick as glass shatters, that's how fast my life changed when Mom was diagnosed with cancer. Her treatments made her lose her appetite. When she lost her appetite, guess what? I found mine.

I ate everything in sight. The thinner Mom got, the more I ate and hoped she'd eat too. I wasn't hungry when I ate. I was nervous about Mom. It seemed like the more treatments she got the sicker and thinner she was. My dad tried to act macho, like she was going to get better. But deep down in my gut, I was afraid she would never get better or look like she used to.

Mom used to be a happy, tall, slim, olive-skinned, beautiful lady. The cancer changed her personality and the way she looked. I didn't even recognize my own mom. It seemed like she was disappearing right before our eyes.

And then she died. I was devastated. She was gone. Like the reading at her burial that said, "Ashes to ashes and dust to dust."

When Mom died, it felt like someone opened up my chest, snatched my heart out, jumped all over it, and then handed it back to me. I ate everything I could. I was out of control.

Now I'm an overweight fourteen-year-old. My height is five feet seven and I weigh a hundred and sixty-three pounds. I have a BMI of twenty-five point five.

There was another reason I overate. It started after Mom's death. I realized that Dad would be the only one who worked and made money. Before Mom got sick, she used to work too, and both my parents made money. So I began to ask myself questions like, "Does Dad make enough money to pay the mortgage? Can he buy us clothes? What about food?"

Then I started to panic. I thought, "Food! Oh no! I'm not going to eat!" I feared that I would not get enough to eat, because Dad wouldn't make enough money.

Before Mom died, every Friday she, Dad, and I went shopping for food. Now that it's only Dad who works, we shop for food once a month. I knew that was because there was not a lot of money. We can't buy all the things we used to buy when Mom was alive. Dad says, "We can't buy extras, only the things we need."

So when it was time to eat, I felt nervous and scared. And what happened was that whenever I went to school or over to someone's house, I'd eat like crazy. My thoughts of not being able to eat at home were real.

At school, there was a nice lady who worked in the cafeteria. She was short and round, and always wore a red-and-white plaid apron. Her short, curly, white hair was tucked under a net. Now this lady knew I did not eat well on the weekends. She noticed that on Mondays when I ate breakfast at school, I ate real fast.

One day she came over to me and said, "John, you ate your breakfast so fast, I wondered if you tasted what you just ate."

I just looked up at her and smiled, so she wouldn't ask any more questions. The next Monday as I ate breakfast, she came over again and said, "Now John, I noticed on Mondays when you eat breakfast, you eat it extremely fast. I don't want to get into your family's business, but I don't believe you get enough to eat on weekends."

I didn't answer, but kept eating.

"Look John, here at school you can eat as much as you want. We have plenty of food here for you. But do me a favor. When you eat, I would like it if you took your time. I do not want you to choke on your food."

As she walked by me, she patted me on the shoulder. I looked into her eyes.

"Now listen, young man, everything is going to be alright, okay?"

"Thanks," I said. I needed to hear that.

When I went into the cafeteria on Mondays, I started to take two breakfasts. But I ate slow and enjoyed my food. The cafeteria lady was so right. My fear of not enough food in my house was real. At that time, all I thought about was where I was going to get my next meal.

To help Dad with our food bill, the lady referred Dad and me to a place where we signed up for food stamps. Dad qualified for them, because he did not make a lot of money. About two weeks later, we got a card to buy food each month.

Now we have enough food in our house. I take my time and eat. Oh and by the way, on Mondays, I still eat two breakfasts, because that cafeteria lady makes the best pancakes I've ever eaten.

Those are my reasons for overeating. I will never get over the loss of my mom, but I've learned how to deal with it better. And I know that overeating won't bring my mom back. I'm ready to lose the weight and become a fly guy again.

I know everybody has a story that explains why they've gained weight or overeaten. Their stories could be social, emotional, academic, or about physical or sexual abuse. Regardless of what it is, or why they've adopted food as their best friend, it's important to address the issues that make them overeat. People need help to really put those issues behind them and live life without being addicted to food.

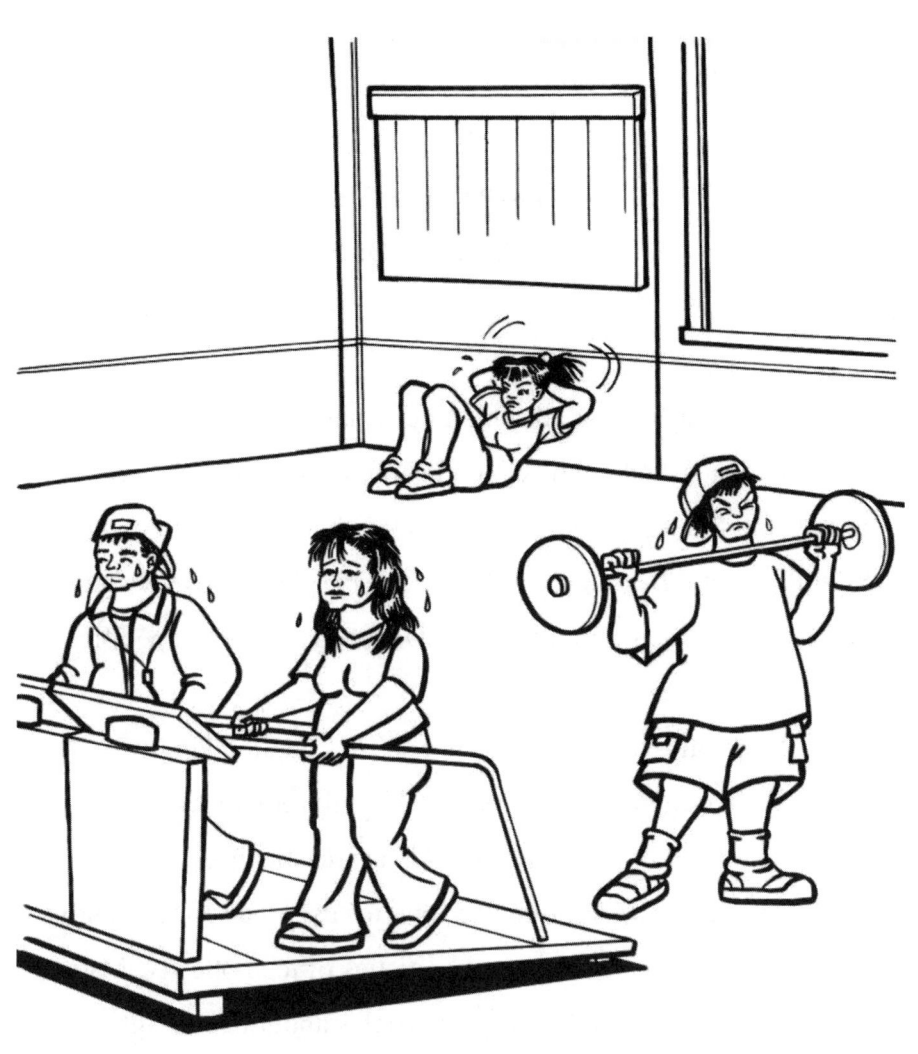

# CHAPTER FIVE
## Let's Get It On!


"Hey guys, do y'all remember what Ms. Sussman said to us?" Davanna asked the next Sunday afternoon. School had started, and the four friends met at Seth's house to do homework and talk about when they would begin their plan to lose weight.

"She told us a lot of things, Davanna. Be more specific, girl," Seth replied.

"She said, 'If you all are not serious about losing weight, you've wasted my time and yours.' Do y'all remember?"

"Now I do," Maritza responded sarcastically.

"Well, she was right. The time for us to be serious is now. We don't want to continue being statistics of teen obesity. My mom and I were online looking up articles about overweight teenagers. We also found and read stories about obesity. One thing we found was a speech by First Lady Michelle Obama. In January 20, 2010, she spoke about America's obese children.

"She said, 'Right now, nearly one-third of children in America are overweight or obese. That is one in three children.

One third of all children today will eventually suffer from diabetes.' She wants to help ensure that children get nutritious meals in school as well as opportunities to exercise, and provide parents with access to healthy, affordable food and clear information about nutrition and exercise."

"When I read her speech, I felt that Mrs. Obama wasn't happy with the number of American children who were overweight or obese. She explained how American children do not eat well. Their schools have not provided them with enough nutritious foods. And the grocery stores in our neighborhoods have not sold us the healthiest foods. Finally, she spoke about how we're not getting off of our butts to exercise on a daily basis. Although she said it in a nicer way, I believe that one of the First Lady's hopes for American children is that we will step on our scales at home, or in school, or at a clinic, and watch the numbers that used to be bigger shrink and get smaller again.

"If we ate healthy foods and exercised, she'd be happy. By being serious about these two things, we would reduce our weight and become healthier Americans. C'mon, y'all, Mrs. Obama's requests are not that hard to do."

"Have y'all realized that the First Lady said some of the same things that Ms. Lemon and Ms. Sussman said?" Maritza replied.

"Yeah," said Davanna. "If I didn't know any better, you'd think all three of them had set us up to lose weight."

"It's like they had a three-way phone conversation," John responded.

"I wouldn't put it past them. You know when educators get together for the same purpose, you can't trust them," Seth said. "No disrespect to you, Davanna, or Maritza, but guess what those three educators also have in common?"

"What's that?" asked Davanna.

"They're all ladies. And guys know that when you've dealt with ladies, sometimes it's like fighting a losing battle. You can't win," Seth concluded.

"Oh really?" Maritza yelled. "Do you want to tell Davanna and me about any more of your thoughts about females?"

"If I were you, Seth, I would not continue that conversation," John said.

"Okay, let's move on. Are y'all ready to lose our weight?" Davanna asked.

Seth, John, and Maritza yelled, "Yeah! You bet we are!"

"Like the old-school singer said, 'Let's get it on,' Davanna sang.

"We've been talking about this for a long time. Let's get started," said John.

"There's no better day than today for starting to change our eating habits and doing daily exercise," said Davanna. "Ms. Sussman said we could use the clinic's scale at the community center to get our true weights, so we should meet at the community center on Mondays. But let's begin by weighing ourselves today. Seth, does your house have a scale we can use? Did everyone bring their notebooks?"

Seth left his room and brought back the scale from the bathroom. One by one the four friends weighed themselves. In their notebooks they wrote their actual weights next to their goal weights.

"There are a lot of ways to report to each other how much weight we've lost. First, we could do it as a group. That means we'd have to publicly report to the group our current and goal weight. Second, we could write down our current and goal weights and keep them to ourselves and just report on our progress. Third, we could choose partners and share our goals with them and lose weight as teams. We could give a reward to the team that loses the most weight. Any of these ways is okay, since our common goal is to lose the weight. Each one of us has to choose the way that's the most comfortable for them."

"I'm good with any one of those options," Maritza replied.

"Me too, I'll go along with the group," Seth said. John nodded.

"Well it seems like none of us have a problem talking to each other about our weight," said Davanna. "My thoughts are that we feel comfortable losing weight as a group and sharing our numbers with each other. Someone tell me if I'm wrong. Y'all know there's no shame in my game. I'll tell how much I weigh in a minute."

"If we lose the weight as a group, we can encourage each other better," said John. "Or give support especially when one of us feels a little down. As a group, we can remind each other not to eat those homemade chocolate chip cookies that just came out of the oven. Do y'all agree?"

"Yeah, he might be right," Maritza said.

"Okay! Is everyone ready to report their true and goal weight?" Davanna yelled.

Before she could say another word, John stepped up.

"My true weight is one hundred sixty-three pounds and my goal weight is one hundred and forty. When I lose these twenty-three pounds of chest-to-waist love handles, I'll be slim and trim again."

"Thanks John," said Seth. "My current weight is one hundred and fifty pounds. My goal weight is one hundred and thirty pounds, so I have twenty pounds to lose. Y'all know that when I lose this twenty-pound stomach, I'll be untouchable."

"That's a coincidence, because I also have twenty pounds to shed," Maritza said. I'm weighing in at a hundred forty pounds, but my goal weight is a hundred and twenty. I can stand to lose twenty pounds of boobs and thighs. But don't get it twisted! I'm still a caramelized beauty, all hundred forty pounds of me. Get it!"

"We're all about twenty pounds from our goal weight, including me," Davanna said. "I wonder, was the food really that good, to put us all about twenty pounds heavier than we want to be?"

The teens looked at each other. Before anyone could answer, Davanna said, "I didn't think so. Well, it's my turn to report my weight. My weight is one hundred thirty-five pounds and my goal weight is one hundred fifteen. I'm already p-h-i-n-e fine, but after I lose twenty pounds I'll have a little less butt and thighs. Beyoncé will have some stern competition. You just wait until I lose this weight, y'all will not know me. Yes, it will be me, the gorgeous one!"

"Hey Davanna, now that we've decided on how we're going to report our weight, what are we going to do to support our weight goals at school and other places?" Maritza asked.

"Well, I've been thinking about that. There are several things we can do. We can start by creating a petition and bringing it to our school district's food program. We'll request that they prepare only healthy foods for lunch and snacks."

"Like what?" Seth asked.

"Okay, let me help y'all. How about salads, chicken wraps, baked fish with steamed vegetables? Raw carrots, celery sticks, sliced apples and oranges? We can also add fruit salads with granola sprinkled on top, spring water, one percent milk, and a hundred percent fruit juices. If these were our only food options at the cafeteria, we wouldn't be tempted to buy cheesy pizza, hot fries, and fried chicken. And we want them to stop selling tuna fish sandwiches that are heavy with greasy mayonnaise, and potato chips, apple pies, and extra large chocolate chip cookies.

"Next, we'll copy the names and addresses off of the vending machines and write each company a letter. We'll leave spaces for as many students as we can get to sign it. We'll ask the companies to remove chips, fried onion rings, cookies, and candies from the machines. We want them to replace the junk food with granola bars, healthy breakfast bars, pretzels, trail mix, and fruit. Then if they don't honor our request, we'll have to take another step and stop buying from the machines. As my mom says, 'Take money out of their pockets.' That'll force the vending machine owners to honor our request. They would rather have some money from selling healthy foods, than no money from selling junk foods.

"We have to be a voice to tell the school district's food program and the vending machine owners that we want them to purchase healthier foods for the students in our school. This will support our weight goals and make Mrs. Obama proud of us too.

"To support our weight goals within the community, we'll have to go to the clinic and get free passes for the wellness programs. Ms. Lemon said she can get us the passes and we can use them to join the community center's aerobics and swim classes. Each class meets two times a week. Aerobics meets on

Mondays and Wednesdays and swim class meets on Tuesdays and Thursdays. That would be four days of physical activities.

"If we're serious about losing weight, on another two days of the week we can take thirty-minute walks around the school track or through the park. If we did that Fridays and Saturdays, maybe on Sundays we should just rest. Do you think we can handle all that?"

"We can do both the aerobics and swim classes if we put our minds to it," John said.

Seth and Maritza nodded.

"We left out one area of our lives," Maritza said.

"What's that?" asked John.

"What do we do when we're home alone and food is calling our names?" Maritza asked. "I've tried to make myself fall asleep so my thoughts of food would go away. But once I'm asleep, I dream about all the goodies in the refrigerator and cabinets. One time a dream made me get up from my bed, and I sleep-walked into the kitchen to satisfy my food cravings. In the kitchen I grabbed a big slice of chocolate cake with chocolate frosting and a chocolate kiss on the top. As I opened my mouth to eat, I woke up and yelled for help, because no one was around to talk me out of shoving the whole damn slice of cake into my mouth. I ask y'all, what's a girl to do?"

"That's real simple," Seth said. "We'll tell our parents about our goal to lose twenty pounds. We'll ask them not to buy or bake chocolate cakes with chocolate frosting with a chocolate kiss on the top. I'm serious. We'll ask our parents to support us with our weight goals. We'll ask them not to buy cake, cookies, and chips. Instead we can ask them to buy fruits, sliced vegetables, yogurts, and granola bars. Do you agree with me, Maritza?"

"Yeah, I guess. I'll see what happens."

"You're so right, Seth," said Davanna. "We should ask to go grocery shopping with our parents. Then we'll be sure that we've picked healthy foods to help us lose weight. In the store we can read the food labels to see how much sugar and salt is in each product. Then we'll look for the correct serving size, the number of calories, and how much fat the food contains before we buy it."

John scratched his head and said, "You know, losing weight is going to be a challenge."

"You're right. But I'll do what I have to do to accomplish my weight goals," Maritza replied.

"What else could we do at home?" Seth said.

"C'mon, Seth!" Davanna said. "We can exercise. There are plenty of exercises we can do at home."

"Like what?"

"Let me tell you just a few. First, we could stop exercising our hands, and I mean lifting our fork or spoon from the plate to our mouths. Instead we should use our hands to get down on the floor and do push-ups and sit-ups. We could walk up and down our stairs three or four times. That would raise our heart rates and we'd burn off calories as we sweat. Another thing to do is press our backs against the wall and slide down toward the floor. As we slide down we'll hold our bodies in a squat position and count to twenty. Then slide back up along the wall to stand up. We'll do that three or four times. Oh, I forgot to tell y'all. The first time, you'll know you're doing it right when the backs of your legs burn like hell. But if we do this every day, the pain will go away.

"The last exercise is to lie on our backs either on the floor or bed. Bring both knees up to your chest and hold them there for a count of ten. Then slowly kick your feet up and lower your legs until they are straight out and level to the top of your body. Remember, as you lower your legs, don't let them touch the floor or bed. Then bring your knees back up to your chest. Continue this exercise three to four times, while you count to ten.

"Those are just some of the exercises we can do at home," Davanna finished.

"So, we do these exercises when we don't go to the gym, swim, or walk?" asked John.

"Correct. These exercises will help us continue to keep moving. Okay! Tomorrow is Monday, the day we begin our workouts. So let's meet at my house. I'll make sure we have some healthy snacks."

Maritza and Davanna left Seth's house together. John stayed behind to talk to Seth.

"I'm so ready to lose this weight, aren't you?" he asked.

"Yeah," Seth said. "I've had it long enough that I've gotten used to it being around. Like, all around my body. It's kept me warm but now it's time to shed the weight. So I'm ready."

"Me too. I can't wait to be tall and slim again."

When Maritza and Davanna had walked a little ways down the street Maritza asked. "Are you ready to start this exercise regimen on a daily basis? I want you to tell me seriously."

"I'm serious as a heart attack," Davanna said. "Girl, I'm tired of what I see in the mirror. I see a beautiful face and a big, big butt. When I lose the weight, I'll feel different when I look in the mirror. And it'll stop the negative things people say around me. Look, after I have time to think about it I really don't care what people say about me. But I don't like dealing with it all the time.

"I have a more important reason for wanting to lose weight. I don't want to be at risk for health problems that come from being overweight. In our health and wellness textbook there's a chapter on obesity that shows different health problems people get from being overweight. It discusses type two diabetes and how that can lead to coronary heart disease, kidney disease, strokes, blindness, or amputation."

"What do you mean, *amputation*?" asked Maritza.

"I mean somebody with this disease can have their toes, feet, legs, arms, fingers, or any other limb cut off, if their diabetes gets out of control."

"Damn, that's deep."

"Yeah, it is. That's why I don't even want to get the disease. One way to prevent it is to not be overweight. But since I am, I have to lose some weight. When I read that chapter, I got scared. Just like you, my thoughts about losing a limb stuck in my head. You know, you can also get high blood pressure from being overweight. High blood pressure already runs in my family. One thing I can do to help prevent these diseases in myself is by losing weight. That's the real reason I want to do this."

"I never looked at it that way. This is serious."

"You're damn right it is," Davanna continued. "I'll tell you a story about a girl I know who was overweight. This is a true story. But after the story, I have to go home."

"Yeah, I heard you. Me too."

"Okay. At school I know a girl who's obese. She's about five feet two and must weigh about two hundred fifteen pounds. She's the picture of teen obesity. The size I never want to be. She's kind of sad. But girl, let me tell you about her.

"She liked to wear these black skin-tight leggings with a fire-engine-red fitted sweater. The sweater was so tight you could count her rolls of fat. You could see the smallest roll sitting underneath her breasts. The next two rolls were larger. The last roll of fat was the biggest one of all. It hung over the top of her black leggings. The tight red sweater did not stretch over her huge butt. Oh, it was sad.

"As she walked down the corridor toward me, I noticed she had on a new pair of sneakers. Now you know how people walk when they have on a new pair of sneakers and they don't want the toe areas to get creases or lines?"

"Yes, I know," said Maritza. "When I have on new sneaks, I'm trying so hard not to mess them up that when I walk I look like I have bad feet."

"You are so right! So, I thought that was the reason the thick girl walked that way. So I said to her, 'You really don't want to put creases in your new sneakers, huh? I can tell by the way you're walking. Ha ha.'

"She said, 'I wish creases in my sneakers was the reason why I walk like this. It's more serious than creases.'

"'What could be more serious than creases in your new sneakers?' I asked her.

"The thick girl said, 'Well, I have type-two diabetes and I have several cuts on my toes.'

"'You've got what?' I said.

"'When you have diabetes, it's dangerous to have cuts anywhere on your feet. The cuts can cause nerve damage in your feet or legs. If they get infected and aren't treated properly, it could get so bad that my feet or legs might have to be amputated. I already had surgery on my feet. Let me show you.'

"When the girl showed me her feet I said, 'Oh snap!' Maritza, her feet looked like something out of a desert. They were so dry and crusty. I asked, 'You mean, you could get those feet, or else your legs, cut off?'

"She said, 'Yeah girl, that's what I mean.'

"'That's deep!' I said. 'So how did you get all those cuts on your feet?'

"'Well, over the summer I wore open-toe sandals,' she said. 'You know I have to be cute.'

"'Yeah, I understand the cute thing.'

"'Being a diabetic, I knew I was not supposed to wear any kind of open-toe shoes because of the risk of getting cuts. But I didn't care! The sandals matched my outfit. So that's how I got the cuts. And that's the reason why I'm walking this way.'

"'How did you get diabetes?' I asked her.

"'It just happened,' she answered. 'I went to see my doctor and she took some blood from my arm and then she put the blood into this machine. When she got the results back she told me I had diabetes and that I needed to address this disease immediately. My mouth dropped open and I just stood there in shock. I took deep breaths through my mouth. I didn't want to believe her. Who'd have thought it was possible to be a fifteen-year-old diabetic? The disease doesn't even run in my family. The doctor broke it down to me.

"'She told me I was a diabetic because of my weight. Because my weight was out of control. She said I had made poor food selections and had not exercised for a long time. Now these bad habits had caught up with me. She said I would need daily insulin shots and that each day I needed to prick my finger with a machine until I drew blood.

"'I told her I wasn't doing that. I said I'd let the school nurse or my mom do it. The doctor told me the drop of blood in the machine would determine my blood sugar level and give me a number that would help determine if my blood sugar level was either too high or low. Based on that number, then I might have to give myself a shot of insulin. I didn't want to stick myself with a needle. I'm not a doctor or a nurse.'" Davanna stopped and looked at Maritza.

"That's deep," Maritza said. "I don't think I could do that."

"I know," answered Davanna. "That girl told me that the doctor showed her how to prick her finger and where to give herself an injection. And she has to do that to herself. The doctor told the girl she needed to get serious about what she ate and how she stayed physically active. If not, her diabetes would only get worse.

"At the end of our conversation, the thick girl said to me, 'Girl, if you don't want to end up like me, you better watch your weight too. You're thick just like I was.'

"I told her about you and Seth and John, and our conversations with Ms. Sussman. I told her how Ms. Sussman gave us information on how to reduce our weight. I told her how we were creating a schedule for exercise. I invited her to join us and thanked her for her story. I told her to keep in touch.

"Maritza, that girl's story could be any one of our stories. She proved to me that type-two diabetes really can happen to a teenager. If I hadn't already decided to lose weight, her story would have made me change my mind." Davanna yawned. "Now that the sandman just flew past my eyes, I'm ready to go to sleep."

"I understand," Maritza whispered. "That's scary."

"I've got to get home now. See you tomorrow for aerobics class."

"Okay, Maritza said. "I think I'm ready." She was still a little anxious. Changing her eating habits and being physically active was new, and she didn't know if she could make it work.

## CHAPTER SIX
## Let's Make It Happen!


On Monday all four teens woke up anxious, but ready to start accomplishing their weight goals. Davanna asked her mom about what going to an aerobics class would be like.

"Do you think it will be too much for me? You know I haven't exercised for a long time. You and Dad are so physically active. What are your thoughts?"

"I think you'll be fine," her mother said. "With any new exercise you must start slow. It takes time to build up your endurance to keep up with the instructor's pace. The instructor will know that you might be slower than other people in the class. You have to remember that a lot of people in the class will have been doing aerobics for years. They already know the workout routine. Over time, you'll be able to keep up with them. So don't worry, I have faith in you. I'm so glad you've decided to take your health into your own hands."

"Mom, I have another question. How am I going to resist the junk food I'm used to eating?"

"It could be difficult. But you will have support from me and your dad. And you'll have lots of support from Maritza, John, and Seth. Don't you all eat lunch at the same time?"

"Yeah."

"So I'm sure you all can help each other do the right thing and not give in to your old eating habits. Don't worry. You can do this. Now go on to school and have a good day. This evening you'll tell me all about aerobics and how well you all did at lunch."

Lunchtime was the first big test for the We Can't Weight Teens. The four friends met in the cafeteria and stood in line.

"Damn, look at the melted cheese and hot pepperoni on that pizza," Davanna said.

"Yeah, you can smell the sauce on it," Maritza replied. "It looks so good."

"Did y'all see those golden brown fries? You can see they just came out of the hot fryer," Seth added.

"C'mon you guys, don't get weak," said John. "This is the first day we pledged not to eat unhealthy foods. Remember, we have to break our old habits and walk right by the junk food." If y'all had just looked down there in the healthy section, you'd see salads with grilled chicken and burritos stuffed with all-natural foods. Let's go to that section and get something that's going to help us."

They walked past the pizza and fries to the section with the healthy food. Each teenager picked up either a salad or burrito.

Davanna, Maritza, and Seth each looked disgusted. It was hard to turn away from the food they were used to eating. John looked resigned.

They headed for the cash registers. On the way they had to pass an area where the desserts were on display. All kinds of cakes, cookies, and brownies were out, just waiting to be picked up. It seemed like there were desserts as far as their eyes could see. At the far end the kids found fruit, sugar-free custards and puddings, and lemon sorbet. Each picked up a healthy dessert, trying not to look at the cakes and cookies.

While they ate they talked about how hard it was to pass up the pizza, fries, cookies, and brownies.

"John, thanks for your support," Davanna said. "If you hadn't been here, one of us may have eaten the wrong food today. I'm so glad we chose to lose weight as a group. This way we'll always help keep one another in check."

"I know that the pizza and fries are unhealthy. But my nose tried to take over," Seth added. "I've trained my mind, but not my nose. I needed your support, John."

"It was hard to get past the unhealthy food," Maritza said. "But those desserts were torture. It was really hard to walk past that brownie with nuts on it. I felt like I was going to get weak."

"No one said this would be easy, and it isn't," Davanna commented.

They ate slowly, concentrating on the taste of their food and chewing carefully. When they were done with lunch, afternoon classes were about to start. They agreed to meet after school and go to Davanna's house before aerobics class.

When the We Can't Weight Teens arrived at Davanna's house, she led them into her kitchen to show them the snacks she had prepared. She had: spring water and seltzer water, carrots and celery sticks, low-calorie salad dressing to dip the vegetables in, a few sliced apples, and reduced-salt pretzels. Each teen looked at the healthy snack choices with disappointment. There were no chips, sodas, or cookies.

"I guess it's better than eating nothing," Seth sighed, and put a few snacks on a small plate. The others followed. Later, when it was time to leave, they changed their clothes and headed for the gym.

"Well, I'm ready as I'll ever be," John said as they walked. "It's time for me to lose weight. Let the exercising begin!"

"I'm ready too," Seth said. "Where's Davanna?"

She had run back into her house and grabbed four bottles of water for the group. She was nervous about going to the gym. What if all the people in the gym were skinny? Would she be able to keep up with the instructor? What if she got short of breath and passed out? Or people laughed at her while she worked out?"

The receptionist at the community center took their passes and directed them to the teen aerobics class in the mirrored room.

The instructor stood in front. She was built. She looked like she could kick somebody's butt. She was muscular and thin, and wore silver spandex tights and a pink sports bra. Her rib cage was stacked with a six-pack of muscles lined up underneath her breasts all the way down to her waist.

Music was pumping over the sound system. Other teenagers were there, lined up and facing the instructor.

Davanna said, "This class doesn't look so bad. What do you think, Seth?"

"I don't know yet. But the instructor is beautiful. If our bodies are going to be built like hers, we've got a lot of work to do."

The instructor came over to the We Can't Weight Teens and said, "This is the first time I've seen you all in my class. This is a high-impact class, and you need to remember you all are going to get through it alright. If you get tired, it's better to walk in place than to sit down. I don't expect that you will keep up with the class, but that's okay. It's your first day. Just enjoy yourself, and over time you will learn my routine."

Then she ran back to the front of the room and faced the class.

"Hi everyone, my name is Joy!" she said. We came here to work our butts off, right? What? I didn't hear anyone answer. We came here to work our butts off, right?"

This time everyone yelled, "Right!"

95

"That sounds better," said Joy.

"She's about to get real busy," said John. "I hope I can keep up with her. I hope I'm ready for this journey."

"Some of you are here for the first time. Welcome! I'll begin slowly to take you through the basic steps. Then I'll speed up gradually. If at any time you can't keep up, get short of breath, or feel dizzy, just move in place. Try not to stop. I'll understand if you slow down. Okay!"

"Did you hear what she said?" whispered Davanna. "Short of breath? Dizzy? Huh, I don't know if I still feel comfortable. I think she's going to exercise us to death."

"Now I want everyone to spread out. Give yourself enough space so that you don't bump into the person next to you. Let's go!"

Joy turned up the music and started by leading them through several stretching exercises to loosen up their muscles. After ten minutes of stretching, the music got even louder and Joy spoke into a microphone attached to her ear so they could hear her over the music. It was hip-hop music that made everybody want to move, even if they didn't know how to dance.

"We'll use a few basic steps through the entire workout in different combinations. We'll work up to a faster pace. Remember, if I'm going too fast for you, just slow down but do not stop. Believe me, I'll understand.

"We do everything in counts of four in this class. Start by sliding to the left four times, and swing your arms to your right. Watch me, like this. Then walk forward four steps. Continue to swing your arms up and down along your sides, one at a time. Like I'm doing. It's kind of like swimming, except you don't bring your arms over your heads. Does everyone get it?"

"Yeah!" the class yelled.

"Next, walk backward four times. Make sure you keep swinging those arms. Got it?"

"We got it."

"I can't hear you!"

"WE GOT IT!" the class screamed.

"C'mon you all, burn those calories! Burn those buns! Keep those arms swinging as you move! Is everyone alright?"

"Yeah!"

"If you ever need to drink some water, go ahead. Just do not stop moving. Okay, now we'll do the same four steps, but this time put your whole body into it and move faster. Are you all ready?"

"YES!"

"Let's go. Right four, left four, front four, back four. Side to side, forward, then back. Side to side, forward, then back. Swing those arms and don't forget to breathe! Breathe, in through your nose and out through your mouth! In through your nose and out through your mouth! Now spread your legs apart and bend into a squat position ten times. Ready, let's go! Down, and up, that's one. Down, and up, that's two. Squat, and up, three. Don't stop, keep squatting. Just a few more."

For forty minutes, Joy led them through exercises. The We Can't Weight Teens found that they could follow the steps pretty easily, but Joy was able to go much faster than they could. Seth got dizzy, so he walked in place until he felt like he could join in again. John needed to drink some water, but as he did so he kept walking like Joy had suggested. Maritza's breathing got short, and that worried her, but she slowed down until she felt better and could keep up again. Davanna lost count sometimes, but Joy was always talking to lead them through what to do. She was embarrassed when she got out of sync with everyone else. But when she looked around no one was looking at her. Everyone was focusing hard on what they were doing. There was no time to pay attention to anything else.

Finally, Joy yelled, "Alright everyone, for the next ten minutes we'll do our cool down! This is at a much slower pace. It's designed to bring your heart rate back down to normal. Let's take it slow. Now reach for the sky, like this. Stretch, and stretch."

Joy turned down the volume and put on slower music. The class moved in slow motion compared to what they had been doing before.

"How does everyone feel? If this is your first time, you've just completed sixty minutes of exercise. Give yourself a great big round of applause."

Almost everyone clapped. Davanna looked at her friends. All of them had wet hair and were covered in sweat from head to toe.

"We made it! We all lived through that hard work out," Davanna panted.

"At first I thought I was going to pass out," Seth said, "because I'm out of shape. But after the first ten minutes, I kind of got into the groove of the music and it didn't feel so bad."

"I felt the same way," John said, breathing hard. "At first I was afraid of losing my breath. Then I slowed down and sipped on the bottle of water. That's when I felt better. After a while, I caught my breath and was able to keep up."

"When we began, my chest felt a little heavy. My breathing was short. Then I said to myself, 'Maritza, you've got to do this. It's for your health. You can't give up, just slow down and you will get through it.' And guess what, I finished! I'm so proud of myself that I can't wait until Wednesday's class."

They walked from the gym back to Davanna's house. They all felt sore in their muscles from the workout. But it wasn't so bad.

During the walk, they discussed their exercise routine.

"Well, tomorrow is Tuesday and we go back to the community center for the swim class. I think it'll be fun. I haven't swum since I was a little girl. How about y'all?" Davanna asked.

Maritza replied, "You know you're right, Davanna. The last time I swam, I was eight years old. As I got heavy I was too embarrassed to put on a bathing suit. So I stopped swimming. But I always loved the water."

"Well, I was never a swimmer," John said. "I can't swim, but always wanted to learn. This is my chance. I know I won't be the most attractive dude in swimming trunks at the pool, but in a few months I will be. You know what? So far I've enjoyed losing weight as a group."

"I couldn't think of a better group to lose weight with," Seth said. "I can't wait for our swimming class so I can jump into the water."

"Let's keep this groove going until we reach our weight goals!" Davanna yelled as they walked up to her house.

They were starved after aerobics class. They ate the last of Davanna's snacks, which tasted good. Then everyone had to go home. Davanna walked them to the door.

"I'll see y'all tomorrow at school. Remember, until we meet again, eat healthy," she said.

Her mom was waiting in the family room to hear about her aerobics class and the first day of eating healthy at lunch. "How did it go?"

"Mom, I never knew that being active was so much fun."

"Are you serious? Or does that mean the aerobics class was not difficult?"

"No, I can't say that. It was difficult, when I started. But it got easier. Joy, the instructor, talked to us new people before class began. She said if we got tired we could just move in place. She said it was okay if we couldn't keep up and that over time we would learn her routines. And she told us to enjoy ourselves.

"So I liked how she made us feel comfortable before we started. Even though I got nervous when she explained what might happen to us while we exercised. But then, when I survived the class, I felt great! I was so proud of myself."

"How did it go at lunch?" her mom asked.

"It felt different at lunch. I wasn't so proud of myself. I just about got weak in the cafeteria and destroyed my weight goal. When I saw all the hot pepperoni pizzas, fries, and desserts, I almost lost it."

"Davanna! Did you eat the junk food?"

"No, but if John wasn't there I would have. He made Maritza, Seth, and me walk past the junk food and go straight to the healthy food area. We could still smell all of the hot oily cheese and fried food, and it smelled so good. We were tempted. But we remembered our goals and only bought healthy food. While we ate we talked about how hard it was to pass by the junk food. It helped to realize how hard it is to break old habits. We all thanked John for being so strong, because the rest of us were so weak."

"Davanna, I'm proud of all four of you. The fact that you all passed on the junk food means that you are all serious about your weight goals. Each one of you deserves praise for sticking to your goals. The first day of any new routine is hard. I'll bet tomorrow will be better. I have so much faith in all of you."

"Thanks Mom," Davanna smiled. She needed to hear that. "It wasn't easy, the aerobics class or lunch. But we got through both. Tomorrow's our first swim class."

"Like I told you this morning Davanna, you'll be fine, honey.

That evening Davanna ate a light healthy supper. She had grilled chicken salad with low-calorie blue cheese salad dressing and iced tea. But in her dreams, she still smelled the hot cheese pizza and greasy fries.

The next day the We Can't Weight Teens met in front of the school building in the morning. They all complained about how their bodies felt.

"When I woke up this morning I was in so much pain, it felt like a herd of football players tackled me," Davanna said.

"I hear you," said John. "I'm still tired. My body hurts too."

"When I watched y'all as you walked, I thought, 'We're all tired,'" added Maritza. "That workout was new to all of us. But in time we'll get used to it. Then we won't be so tired or ache so much."

"I sure hope you're right," Seth said. "I slept like a bear in hibernation after Joy's workout. This morning I was in pain too. But I worked out so hard that I earned my sleep."

"I thought we all did one hell of a workout, and our pain proves it. Well, enough of the complaining. Let's get to class. Make sure y'all do your homework, so we can get to the pool on time."

Seth had complained to his mom about his aching muscles. She figured his friends felt the same, so she met them in front of the school at the end of the day. She drove them over her house for a healthy snack before swim class. In the car, they told Mrs. Bernstein about their weight goals and how they were changing what they ate.

"That's great," she said. "I'm glad you all have decided to do what's best for your health. I want to support you all, and I've got healthy snacks waiting at home. We have yogurt, fresh fruit, pretzels, air popped-popcorn, all-natural juice, and bottled water. That should hold you over until you get home."

The teens ate their snacks at Seth's house, and when it was time for swim class, Mrs. Bernstein drove them to the community center. They changed into their swim gear in the locker rooms. Davanna had on her one-piece orange bathing suit. Maritza wore her royal blue skirt swimsuit. Seth wore his black-and-white striped trunks, and John wore his black trunks.

They met in the pool area. None of them were ashamed to be standing around in their swim gear, even when they walked by guys with muscled chests and girls shaped like Barbie. For the We Can't Weight Teens, their physical appearances had become something they didn't worry about as much, because they had decided to lose weight.

A group of teenagers waited at one end of the pool for the class to start. They stood around a man and a woman wearing swimsuits.

"Hi everyone, my name is Malique," said the man. "I'll be your lifeguard." Malique had olive-colored skin with green eyes and black curly hair. His orange swimsuit hugged his muscular legs.

"Ooh girl! He's gorgeous. He can save me anytime," Davanna whispered to Maritza.

"He does look good," Maritza replied. I think we've been in the house with food too long. Look at what we've missed. He's a lot of man."

"I'm going to love to swim here," Davanna giggled.

"Me too, girlfriend."

The woman introduced herself as Stacey, the swim instructor. She was tall and thin, and tan from head to toe. Her long blonde ponytail hung down to her narrow waist.

For John it was love at first sight. Right then he was sure he was going to learn how to swim, even if it killed him.

"All I need is a tender touch and guidance from her," he whispered to Seth. "I'll swim like a fish before you can count to three."

"C'mon John, stop tripping. Stacey's job is to teach people how to swim. That's what's important today."

Malique blew his whistle. "The pool has safety rules. Anybody who wants to swim in the deep end of the pool must take a swim test first. This is required! You have to swim from one side of the five-foot area to the other." He pointed to the side of the pool, which had a big number five on it. "Then you have to tread water for about one minute. Once you pass, you can swim in the deep end, which is the eight-foot to ten-foot area." He pointed again to the numbers on the side of the pool. "That's the end where I sit. Understand?"

"Yes," everyone replied.

Davanna, Seth, and Maritza ran over to the five-foot area. One at a time they swam from one side to the other and back. Then they showed Malique how they could tread water for a minute. He told them they passed and that they were allowed to go into the deep end.

In a soft voice, Stacey spoke to the kids who hadn't taken or passed the test. "The rest of you need to stay in the three-foot area. Please don't go under the red-and-white floating line stretched across the five-foot mark."

She picked up a bullhorn and spoke through it, which made her louder. "If anyone is interested in learning how to swim, I teach a lesson in the three-foot area with floating devices. Just grab a floater and step into the pool. You all can join the other beginners who are lined up along the wall!"

John grabbed a floater, which was a big piece of plastic Styrofoam, and got into the pool and stood near Stacey. He was happy to have a reason to get next to her.

"To begin, everyone put one hand on each of the two corners of the floater." Stacey demonstrated. "Like this. Now put your backs against the wall of the pool. Lean back. Then you're going to push off with one of your feet. When you float away from the wall, keep your feet side by side. You're going to glide until your feet drop down in the water. Watch and I'll demonstrate."

She showed them the correct way to glide. "This is called floating and it's the first stage of learning how to swim. When you swim, your body is floating through the water. Don't be afraid, I'll have each one of you push off and glide, one at a time. I'll stand right next to you."

John was afraid to try. He'd never done it before. But with Stacey beside him, for a second it seemed like anything was possible. When it was his turn, as soon as he pushed off, his legs fell to the bottom of the pool. He was embarrassed.

Stacey put her hand on his shoulder. "That was a great first try. Don't get discouraged. Learning how to float takes practice. But don't give up. You'll need to try several times before you get it. Remember, practice makes perfect. Soon you'll be floating on your own."

Stacey moved on to help the next student. John tried again and again. Stacey wasn't looking at him anymore, and he wanted her attention. He gripped the floater tightly and pushed off from the wall as hard as he could. He was floating!

He yelled, "Hey Stacey, I did it. I did it, I floated!"

She came back over to him and congratulated him. "Great! Now that you've done that, let me show you the correct way to kick your feet."

She showed him first, and then he tried it. Before he knew it, he had traveled across the pool. When he got to the side he stopped and yelled, "I can float across the pool! I floated by myself!"

Davanna, Seth, and Maritza heard John yell. They climbed out of the deep end and hurried over to congratulate him.

"I knew you could do it," Davanna said. "Soon you'll be able to swim. The hardest part is behind you. Once you can float, you can swim."

"I couldn't have done it without help from Stacey. She's the greatest."

Davanna noticed the gleam in John's eyes and a smile on his face. "You have a crush on Stacey, don't you?" she whispered.

John just smiled.

When John's swimming lesson was over, his three friends joined him in the three-foot area. They had spent the time swimming laps in the deep end the way Malique had told them to, from the ten-foot marker to the five-foot marker and back.

"Okay now you have free time," Stacey yelled. "You can practice what you've learned or just have some fun in the water."

All four played water tag. As they played they were hardly even aware they were exercising. Davanna, Seth, and Maritza swam across the pool easily, as if they were sharks. John continued to use the floater. He stretched his arms in front of him and kicked his feet. Soon he was moving across the pool very well. They stayed in the water until Malique blew his whistle to signal that swim hour was over.

"I had an awesome time," panted Maritza as they walked toward the locker rooms.

"I never had that much fun in the water before, because I was always scared," said John.

"I had so much fun. I thought I had lost my swimming skills, but I hadn't," Davanna said.

"That was great!" Seth added. "The water was warm and it felt good. I had a ball."

They changed clothes and went outside. Mrs. Bernstein was waiting for them in the car. "How was it?" she asked.

As usual, Davanna began. "It was the greatest, Mrs. Bernstein. I thought I'd forgotten how to swim. But when I went into the water, my swimming skills came right back to me. I was like a fish."

"Hey Mom, when I dived into the water, I felt like a shark swimming hard. It was so natural," Seth told her.

"Maritza?"

"Mrs. Bernstein, I'm going to be honest. I was scared because I hadn't been in the water for a long time. But when I got into the pool, it was like I had never taken a break from swimming."

"What about you, John?" Mrs. Bernstein asked.

"Well, it was my first time, but I floated across the pool like a seal. And there was a beautiful instructor named Stacey. She made my day. I can't wait until Thursday's class."

"So I take it everyone enjoyed themselves?" Mrs. Bernstein asked.

"Yes!" they all said in unison.

Mrs. Bernstein dropped everyone off at their homes and then took Seth home for a healthy dinner, homework, and bed.

Wednesday was the third day of the healthy eating and exercise regimen. That morning everyone arrived at school feeling more tired and sore than the day before.

"I don't know about y'all, but I'm exhausted. My body aches from aerobics and then swimming. Now it's Wednesday and we'll have to go back to aerobics. I'm so tired it felt like I ran from monsters in my sleep for two whole nights."

"You're so right, Davanna. I'm exhausted too." John sighed. "I had a lot of fun in the water. It was great. And I kicked so much that I forgot it was exercise. But today I can feel it. Every muscle in my body aches."

"My mom woke me up this morning because I slept like a dead man in a coffin," Seth said. "It seemed like I'd just gone to sleep. But in reality, I went to bed at nine last night and mom woke me up at six a.m. Those nine hours of sleep felt more like an hour."

"I'm so knocked out I haven't had time to get online, connect on Facebook, or play computer games," Davanna said. "But that's the point of exercise, right? We're supposed to be exhausted. Remember what Ms. Sussman said. We're using muscles we haven't used in a long time. Plus, we burned calories."

"I haven't had time to sit at the computer or watch TV eating a snack," Maritza said.

"That means being physical has worked," Davanna said. "When we got home we were so tired all we could do was eat a small meal, take a shower, and go to bed. I'll bet that when we go to the clinic and weigh ourselves, we'll all have lost weight."

"Like y'all, I'm so, so tired," said Maritza. "When I woke up today every muscle and bone in my body ached. But I

remembered that we'd agreed to go to aerobics on Mondays and
Wednesdays, and swimming class on Tuesdays and Thursdays.
And we also said we'd walk thirty minutes on Fridays and
Saturdays. So I understood that this pain would be with me for a
while."

"Let's not forget: no pain, no gain," Davanna replied.
"After school, we'll go to John's house before our aerobics class.
So we'll meet here in our usual spot, okay?"

Lunch in the cafeteria was getting a little easier. They were
going directly to the healthy food area and choosing meals from
there. They could still smell the fries and the pizza, and they still
saw the delicious desserts on their way out. But when one person
felt a little temptation, the others helped remind them of their goals
and how to accomplish them. They wanted to eat in the cafeteria
like other students. But if the temptation was too great, they knew
they could follow Ms. Sussman's suggestion and buy lunch boxes
and bring their own lunches. And after school, they'd have snacks
at one of their houses.

John promised that he had prepared a delicious snack for
his friends after school. And when they got to his house that
afternoon he said, "Y'all are going to love this. I made small
ground turkey burritos this morning. And there's some lettuce and
tomatoes in the fridge if you want that. There's also low-calorie
dressing and flavored water in the ice chest."

"I sure hope the water is cold, because by the time we finish aerobics, I'll be thirsty and could use a cold drink," Seth said.

"Hey John, these are mighty good," Maritza muttered as she chewed.

"Thanks I tried to make them like my dad does. He makes a mean burrito."

When they finished their snacks, they changed into their workout clothes. When it was time to go to the gym for class, they each took a bottle of flavored water and walked together.

In the community center, as they walked to the room where the teen aerobics class was held, they passed a young man who was tall, handsome, and built. He had muscles everywhere. His gray T-shirt hugged every muscle in his chest. His waist was small and he had the right amount of junk in his trunk.

"He's fine as hell," Davanna whispered.

"He sure is," Maritza replied.

John and Seth noticed the girls' reactions and studied the young man.

"He looks like he lives in the gym," said John.

"If we came here as much as he did, we'd look like him too," Seth said.

The young man walked over to Seth and John. "My name's Joshua and I'm a physical trainer. Whenever you guys are ready to look like I do, meet me in the large gym. I can help you both build some muscles if you want."

"One day we'll take you up on that offer. But right now, we have a class," John said.

"Thanks for the offer though," mumbled Seth.

When they got to class Joy was all ready to go, with her microphone on and the music blasting. "Today we're going to do a Zumba workout," she announced.

"What in the heck is that?" Davanna whispered.

"A Zumba workout matches different Latin music rhythms with easy-to-follow dance steps. We use steps from dances like the merengue, salsa, reggaeton, and cumbia. You will sweat your butts off and burn a lot of calories. Just follow me and you'll pick it up easily. We'll start with stretches to loosen you up."

After ten minutes of stretches, Joy turned up the Latin music. "Remember, if you can't keep up, it's okay. But if you need to rest, don't stop moving, Just walk in place. Are we ready?"

"Yeah!" the class shouted.

"Well, let's go!"

The teens watched Joy and did what she did. They twisted their waists and danced their feet from left to right. They clapped as they circled the gym. They jumped up and down to the beat. They moved so much that sweat ran down their faces and dampened their clothes. The steps weren't hard to figure out. They were dancing!

After forty minutes Joy yelled, "Okay everyone, get some water. As you drink, don't stop moving. Walk in a big circle."

A minute or two passed. Joy spoke into her microphone. "Okay, we're bringing your heart rates down slowly. We'll do some cool down stretching. Remember, you should always cool down after intense exercise."

For the last ten minutes of class, Joy led them through several stretches that helped their muscles and lowered their heart rates. Then she taught them how to find their own heart rates. They each pressed two fingers to their necks and found the carotid pulse. They walked around in circles and watched the big clock on the wall. For one entire minute, they counted the number of pulses under their fingers. Joy had each person call out their number. Everyone continued to walk around in circles until Joy was satisfied that the numbers were low enough. Only then did she dismiss the class.

"Now that was intense," Davanna said as they walked out of the room.

"But fun," John replied.

"I've never had that much fun exercising," added Maritza.

Seth said, "Before this week I've never had any fun exercising. But today I danced so hard I forgot we were exercising."

"And we're all drenched! We each need to go home and take showers," Davanna said.

They agreed to meet at Maritza's house the next day before the second swim class, and everyone headed home. They showered, ate, told their parents about Zumba, and went to bed early. Three days in a row of exercise! The We Can't Weight Teens were proud of themselves.

On Thursday they met in front of school before first period. Everyone was moving slowly.

"How's everyone doing?" Davanna asked. "It's a beautiful day, right?"

John and Seth just grunted. Both of them were too tired to speak.

"Hey Davanna, I feel great, even though Joy worked the hell out of us yesterday. Can you two guys speak or does the cat have your tongues?"

"No Maritza, I can speak and the cat does not have my tongue. But I am so tired," Seth answered.

Davanna asked, "John, is your day beautiful?"

"The only beautiful thing about today is that we get to go swimming after school and I'll be close to Stacey," he muttered.

"What about the actual swim lesson?" Seth asked.

"What lesson? When I see Stacey, I forget about the lessons."

"Okay, don't get it twisted. Stacey's job is to teach you how to swim. Not for you to fall in love with. Don't let her

gorgeous body make you forget you're in the water and go under!"
Davanna laughed as the bell rang.

In the afternoon as they walked over to Maritza's mom's
house they talked about how things had been at school during the
week.

"Believe it or not, I thought my grades and homework
would go down," Davanna said, "because of all the time we're
spending at the community center. But guess what? My grades are
higher than before. Isn't that funny?"

"I don't think so, since we're being healthier," Maritza
said. "It makes sense that exercise could help make my grades
healthier too. I can focus better on my homework. What about your
grades, guys?"

"I didn't really notice, but now that you ask you're right.
My grades went up too," John answered.

"Mine too. They went up just like a chairlift up a ski
mountain."

"It's not just the physical activity that's a new positive
thing for us."

"What else," asked Seth?

"Well, we get off our butts and go to the community center
four days a week. We see new people and learn new things. We get
out of the house on a daily basis. Also, we're eating healthy meals
and snacks."

"We haven't sat in front of our computers on Facebook or anything," said Maritza. "Or played computer games with a bag of chips sitting next to us. If computers had feelings, mine would feel neglected. I've only used mine for research or homework this week."

"You're right! We're too exhausted to do anything else," Seth said.

"Now we come in from the community center, turn on our computers, and wait for them to power up. Within that small amount of time, we're asleep. My parents are supporting me too, by eating healthier suppers at night," Seth added.

"Do y'all know one of the most positive things that happened to me?" John asked.

"No, I don't. But I'm sure you're going to tell us," said Davanna.

"I've met that fine swim instructor, Stacey," John replied.

"Speaking of fine, what about that lifeguard Malique?"

"Yeah girl, he sure is fine," Maritza giggled.

"Okay, snap out of it!" Seth said. "Another positive thing is that I'm going to bed at a reasonable hour. When I get home from the community center, I'm too tired to stay up too late. Also, none of us have been late for school because we haven't overslept. That means our bodies are really responding to this new stuff."

"Y'all are going to love my snacks," Maritza said as they walked up to her front door. "I made some Spanish rice and bean tacos with spicy sauce. I also have some all-natural mango juice."

"I've never tasted mango juice," John said.

Maritza led the way to the kitchen and brought out the snacks.

"Umm, these tacos are tasty," John said. "And I like the mango juice. It's different."

"Different, but good. I'm going ask my mom to buy some," Seth replied.

When they finished they headed out toward the community center for their second swim lesson. They changed in the locker rooms and entered the pool area.

The first person who caught John's eye was that fine Stacey. He walked up to her and said, "Huh-hi, Stacey." He was nervous and he stuttered a little. "How was your day?"

"My day was fine, sweetheart, how was yours?"

"If it was bad, you've just changed it," he replied.

Stacey smiled. As John walked over to the three-foot area of the pool, he grinned the whole way. His friends were a little disgusted at the way he acted silly whenever Stacey was around. But then Davanna and Maritza noticed Malique. The disgust on their faces melted into smiles.

"Hi Malique," they both said in playful voices.

"What's up ladies, are you both ready to swim?" His smile was perfect.

"Yes we are," they giggled as Malique kept walking.

Seth groaned. "I don't believe it. Y'all need to get a grip and not lose your damn minds when you see people in swimsuits. What the hell is wrong with y'all? I thought we came here to swim, not fall in love."

Malique blew his whistle, which meant the swim hour was starting. Davanna, Seth, and Maritza went to the ten-foot area and John went to the three-foot area. In the deep end, Malique instructed the teens to swim their laps. In the shallow end, Stacey started the beginners' lesson.

"You need to learn to take air in and blow it out as you swim," she said. "Lay the right side of your face on top of the water. Like this." She showed them how she breathed in air through her mouth, then held her breath and put her face into the water. Finally, she showed them how to blow the air out into the water. Everyone practiced until they mastered these steps.

"I know it seems strange," Stacey said. "But it's one of the most important parts of swimming." She walked around to watch each student and make sure they did the breathing exercise correctly. "John, let me see you do it."

John was thrilled to have her individual attention. He took his time. He laid the right side of his face on the water. He breathed in air and then turned his face into the water and blew it out. Then he took his head out of the water.

"Great job, John! You'll be a swimmer in no time."

John gave her a big smile.

When the lesson was over, they had a half-hour for free swim. The four friends met in the three-foot area and played volleyball in the water over a floating net.

When swim hour was over, and they had changed and were leaving the community center, John told the others about how he'd learned to breathe in the water. The other three talked about how many laps they swam. Again, they had had a lot of fun exercising.

"Tomorrow's Friday," Davanna said. "That means it's been almost one week of being physically active. The time has come for us to weigh ourselves. We've had a lot of fun, but our primary goal was to lose weight. So tomorrow we'll find out how the aerobics and swimming have helped with our goals this week. Let's weigh ourselves before we take our thirty-minute walk. Okay?"

Everyone agreed.

On Friday the teens went to the community center to use the scale.

"I remember you all," the receptionist said after they asked her where to go. "Ms. Lemon and Ms. Sussman gave you permission to use the scale. I've seen you here every day this week. Good for you."

She pointed the way to the scale. They all stood around it, looking it up and down as if it were their enemy.

"Well, the moment of truth has come," said Davanna. It's time to get weighed to see how much we lost. Is everyone ready?"

They looked at each other. Each one of them feared what the scale would tell them. They were nervous as hell. Davanna had sweaty hands. Both Seth and Maritza had beads of sweat on their foreheads. The back of John's T-shirt was wet.

"Okay everyone, who's first?"

Seth stuck out his chest, pulled his shoulders back, and walked to the scale. He looked confident. "I'll go first."

He stood on the scale and watched at the numbers. "I'm rocking it!" he yelled. "I lost six pounds. That's great! I began at one hundred fifty pounds. I went down to one hundred forty-four. Now I only have fourteen pounds to lose to get to my goal."

Everyone clapped for Seth.

"I was going to wait and be last, but I'm too excited. I can't wait," Davanna said.

She stepped on the scale hoping that the numbers would be below 135 pounds. When she saw them she screamed as loud as she could. "Oh snap! I lost five pounds. No for real, I lost five pounds! I'm at one hundred thirty pounds. Damn I'm good! I got fifteen more pounds to lose. Just fifteen more to go." Davanna was so happy she danced around the room.

"Can I go next? Can I, John?" Maritza asked.

"Sure, ladies before gentlemen. I can wait," John replied.

Maritza looked at the scale and put one foot on it. But before she put her other foot on, she thought about something she did the night before. She took her foot of the scale. "John, if you want to go next, you can."

"Why, what are you afraid of?" John asked. "You've eaten healthy food and exercised daily. What's wrong?"

"Well, last night there were chocolate chip cookies at home. I knew I wasn't supposed to eat them. But…they kept calling my name. So I gave in and ate a couple."

"I think you'll be alright," John told her. "As long as the chocolate chip cookies you ate only happened once. Remember, you've exercised and swum your butt off. So go on, girl. Step on the scale, you'll be fine."

Maritza stepped on the scale. When she saw the number she began to cry tears of joy. "Even though I cheated, I still lost seven pounds! When we began I weighed one hundred forty pounds. Now I weigh one hundred thirty-three. I was so guilty because I ate the cookies. Guys, I promise I won't cheat again. After I ate them I felt like I let you all down. You can bet it won't happen again."

The others gave Maritza a group hug. "Anyone can slip every once in a while," Seth said. "It's okay."

"John, it's your turn," Maritza whispered.

He stepped onto the scale. "Huh! I knew it! I lost eight pounds!" he yelled. "At first my weight was one hundred sixty-three pounds. Now it's one hundred fifty-five pounds." John was so excited that he ran around the room and got out of breath. "We did it! We all lost weight! I knew we could do it. I'm so excited!"

He stopped running and looked at his friends. "Hey y'all, let's give ourselves a big round of applause. We each lost five pounds or more after our first week."

"Yes!" Davanna yelled. "And have y'all noticed, we've been so busy with healthy eating and being active that we forgot about our old best friends?"

"What best friends?" Maritza asked. They all stared at Davanna. They thought as hard as they could to figure who these best friends were.

"See, you forgot junk food, candy, cookies, pizza, fries, and soda," Davanna replied. "Your old best friends."

The others laughed as hard as they could.

"Only you could think to say something like that, Davanna. Only you," Seth chuckled.

"Hey Davanna! We didn't lose our best friends," Maritza yelled.

"What do you mean? We stopped eating junk food and all of the other things that are unhealthy. Did I miss something?"

"No, but if you look around, you can see that other people still have them as their best friends."

"I know you're smart, Maritza, but how can you tell?"

"Just look around at school and in the cafeteria. There are still plenty of people who eat junk food for lunch and snacks. They don't pass the hot pepperoni pizza, fries, or dessert like we do. Those are the teens who ask, 'Is that pizza and fries still hot? If they're cold, I'll wait until you fix more.' Remember, we used to ask those questions of the cafeteria staff when we ate unhealthy food."

"Yeah, as long as we continue to eat healthy food and exercise, we won't be one of those people anymore," said John.

"I agree. But let's remember, it's going to be hard for them to pass the junk food area of the cafeteria, because it was hard for us." Seth added.

"It's hard to break old eating habits. But once you set a goal to eat healthy and exercise, it gets easier," Davanna replied. "We'll help them if they ask. Do y'all remember when people looked down at us, because we were overweight?"

"Yeah, like that skinny couple at the beach, who called us fat asses? That will never ever happen to us again," Maritza said. Her face twisted up as she remembered it. "I think that couple's swear was the final insult for us, because right after that we decided to change our lifestyles."

"Remember how Davanna was so pissed that she called the clinic to get us help with being teased?" asked Seth.

"Just think, we showed up there and learned we were overweight," John said.

"That whole scene was horrible. Can you imagine how many other people our age are going through the same thing?" Davanna asked.

"It's no fun at all," said Maritza, her mouth twisting again as she remembered her negative feelings that day on the beach.

"Since we've all lost five pounds or more, how about we continue the same thing we did this week for another six weeks?" asked Davanna. "Maybe by then we'll hit our weight goals. Then we can decide what we need to do after that. What do y'all think? Remember how Ms. Sussman told us, 'While your bodies are adjusting to its new size, you might gain a little weight back before you start losing it again. That's normal. Also, you might find that you'll need to do more exercise to keep your new size than you did to lose it.'"

"I'm so tired," Maritza moaned.

"But you've lost weight. Look at you. You can't forget about being teased, and what Ms. Sussman taught us. C'mon girl, the healthy food and exercise is worth being tired. And to help you get through the next six weeks, just think about that fine Malique in those orange swim trunks. That should help," Davanna reminded her.

Maritza's frown turned into a smile. "Okay, okay, I'm in for another six weeks. But let's take it six weeks at a time."

"Count me in too," John replied.

"You know I'm down," Seth replied.

"So we'll continue our routine for the next six weeks. We had a huge success this week. Let's give ourselves a hand."

Everyone clapped and yelled.

"So is everyone happy?" Davanna asked.

"Yeah, we are!" said Seth.

"Are y'all sure?"

"Yeees, we're sure." Maritza was suspicious.

"Because I have to remind you of something."

"And what is that?" John asked.

"Today we start our thirty-minute walks around the track or through the park," Davanna replied.

She laughed as her friends' smiles turned to frowns.

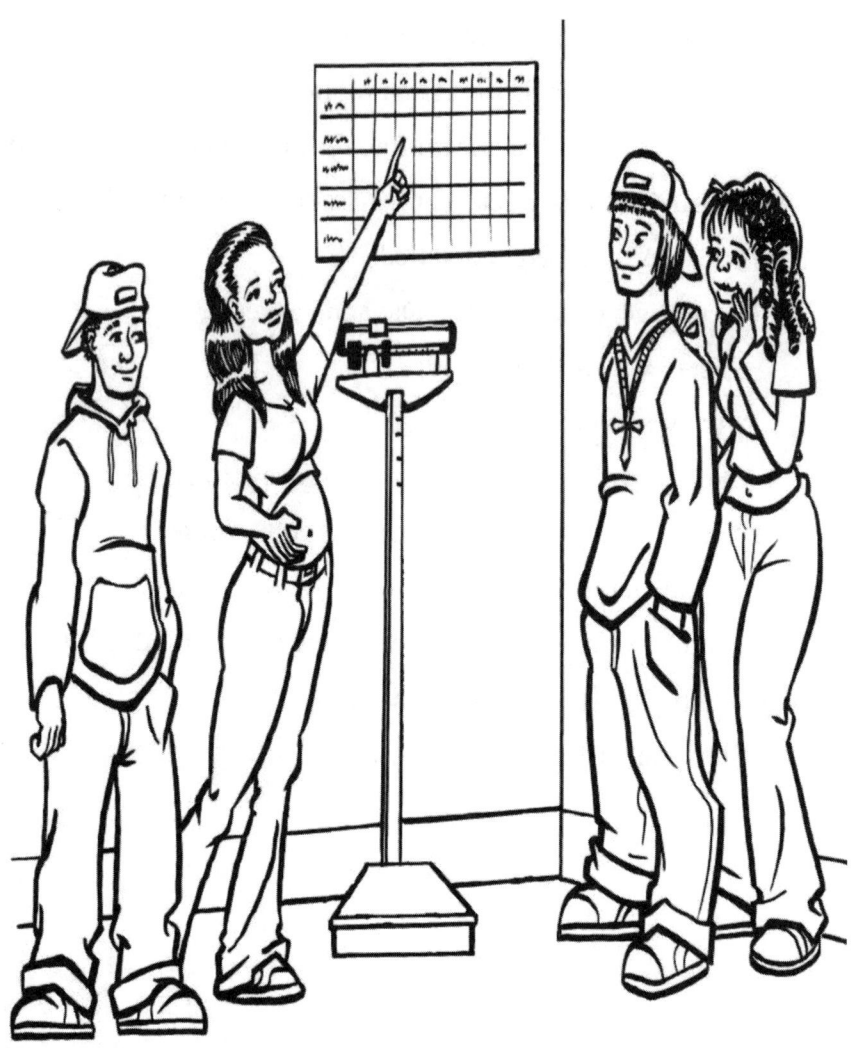

## CHAPTER SEVEN
### We Made It!

After an additional six long weeks, through all the sweat and silent tears, each of the We Can't Weight Teens accomplished their weight goals.

Davanna had started at 135 pounds before Ms. Sussman taught them that healthy eating and physical activities would equal weight loss. Ms. Sussman was right. After six more weeks Davanna weighs 115 pounds. She lost 20 pounds.

When Maritza began her new daily regimen, she weighed 140 pounds. Her final weigh- in was 118. She lost 22 pounds.

Initially, Seth weighed 150 pounds. He got his weight down to exactly 130 pounds. He lost 20 pounds.

John started by weighing 163 pounds. His weight dropped to 140 pounds. He lost 23 pounds.

All four teens now know that changing what they ate and how they exercised allowed them to accomplish their weight goals. Even though they lost the weight they wanted to lose, they continue to eat health food and exercise daily so that they can maintain their goal weights.

The teens still go to the community center for aerobics classes on Mondays and Wednesdays. They still attend swim classes on Tuesdays and Thursdays. They continue their thirty-minute walks on Fridays and Saturdays. Their muscles aren't sore anymore. They feel great!

All four friends believe the most important part of their weight loss was the day they accepted being overweight.

"Knowing I was overweight made me realize I needed to change my lifestyle," Davanna said to her friends one day as they walked around the school track. "And now, healthy eating and daily exercise is my way of life. I wouldn't have it any other way. I lost weight because I changed these two major areas in my life.

"In the past, we thought about trying different things to make us lose some weight. Maybe we'd stop eating sugar, or salt, or we exercised sometimes. Some people try diets when they're overweight. My doctor told me that for a short period of time, the diets seem to work. But after a diet stops, the weight can come right back. After a diet it's easy to go back to old habits that gain weight."

"I did that," said John. "The old habits started up when I ate a little bit of the unhealthy food that we weren't supposed to eat. Food like pizza, fries, and soda. When I weighed myself, the scale didn't go up very much. So I added cookies, chips, and pieces of pie. I got on the scale and it did not lie. I got heavier and heavier. At some point I'd say, 'Oh well, I'm already big,' and eat two more pieces of chocolate cake. Am I right, y'all? Has that happened to you?"

"Amen, you are so right."

"Yes, it happened to me."

"When we ate the chocolate cake without feeling any guilt, that meant we didn't care anymore about our size. We accepted that we were big and that was that," Seth added.

"Sure, you're right," said Maritza. "At that point in time we'd accepted the weight and became comfortable with it. And remember how long it took us to create those unhealthy habits? It took even longer to change them into healthy ones."

"Ditto, you're all right," said Davanna. "Now we've got past those unhealthy ways and accomplished our weight goals, we can maintain our weights where we want them to be. So I'm excited. You know what? I'd like to use the knowledge we've gained to support and advise other teenagers who struggle with being overweight."

"I agree," Maritza said.

"That's great," said Seth. "Let's tell them what we learned."

"Here's my advice to whoever will listen," John said. "To lose weight, you must change what you eat and start an exercise routine. These changes will not be quick or easy. For us, it took time and was difficult. But we hung in there. With help from each other and from the neighborhood clinic, we were able to change our habits. Then we lost weight."

"John's right," Davanna said. "Our unhealthy eating and exercise habits didn't develop overnight. So healthy habits will take some time. Once we've made up our minds to lose weight and started healthy eating and daily exercise, my interest in unhealthy food started to disappear. Especially when I look back at the amount of time and energy we put into our changed habits."

"I remember that first time we went to weigh ourselves to see if we'd lost weight," said Maritza. "I was afraid to get onto the scale, because I had eaten some cookies the night before. I felt guilty and bad, since I believed I had let the rest of you down. We all worked so hard and I cheated by eating the cookies in a few minutes of weakness. I didn't just cheat myself by doing that. I cheated the group.

"So I would suggest to other teens that if they decide to lose weight, it helps to get a few friends to lose weight together. For us, we had each other's backs through the whole process. If one of us didn't take the steps we agreed on, we would have had to answer to the other three people in the group. That was good pressure."

"Here's what I would say to other teens who want to lose weight," Davanna said. "You have to understand that losing weight is a 'you thing.' You are losing weight for *you*. Not for your parents, your friends, or your doctor. My doctor showed me a study in a magazine from Shaw University. It says that 'African-American women between the ages of twelve and nineteen are nearly sixty percent more likely to be overweight. They are less likely to eat fruits, vegetables or whole grains. Also, they are less likely to be physically active than white women in the same age group.'

"Being African-American, that study shocked the heck out of me. My chances of being overweight were documented by some doctors. They all knew about it and I didn't. Go figure! I had to do something so that I would not be one of the sixty percent. I had to make a conscious decision to lose weight.

"This is how I knew it was a 'me decision.' For many years, my parents bought low-fat milk and ice cream. When they cooked, they were careful about the amount of sugar in the food. Sometimes they used sugar substitutes. I ate everything that I was supposed to eat when I was at home, and we ate healthily. But when I went to school, or over to other people's houses, I would pig out on junk food. I did 'sneak eating.' Everything that I couldn't eat at home, I ate somewhere else. Each year when I had my physical examination, my doctor would say with a puzzled look on her face, 'Davanna, you weigh a lot more than you weighed last year.'

"Each year I would just look in the other direction, as if I didn't even hear her. Because I knew my parents were waiting for my answer too. They could not figure out why I continued to gain weight. They had medical tests done on me. They tested my blood, my organs, and my thyroid. But all of the results were normal. So they got suspicious.

"They would say, 'Davanna eats the right foods at home. And we don't give her extra money to buy junk food at school. Something is going on here.' Yeah, they were right. The key words were 'at home.' They realized I was sneak eating. They found out like detectives. When I went to sleep, they checked my book bag and found all kinds of candy and cookie wrappers. So they knew I bought food with the money I did have. They called my friends' parents and found out that I ate chips, cookies, and candies at other people's houses.

"They preached to me like a preacher on a pulpit in church. They helped me realize that when I did my sneak eating, the person I cheated most was me.

"My parents did lots of things to try and help me lose weight. They got even more strict about food in the house and stopped having anything close to junk food at home. We never went to restaurants for burgers and fries. When they drove us by one of those fast-food restaurants, they made sure to drive by fast. My brother and I couldn't even smell the food we went by so fast.

"Mom prepared homemade desserts to control the amount of sugar in each serving. It only takes a little sugar or honey to make something taste sweet. She also took me on walks around the pond and purchased a membership to the gym for me. Yeah, I lost

133

a little weight now and then, but most things my parents tried didn't work. And the reason why is that I was not ready to lose the weight, even though my parents wanted me to. I would tell teenagers that you lose weight anytime *you* want to. You can only lose weight for *you*."

"That's true," said Seth. "Anyone who loves you can try to get you to lose weight, but it doesn't work until you are ready to change your lifestyle. Once you've changed your eating and exercise habits, you have to continue with your goal even when you don't want to."

"There were several reasons why I was able to lose twenty pounds," said Davanna. "First, I realized I wanted to lose the weight for me. Second, I was tired of all the fat names I was called. When people approached me, they looked at me with disgusted expressions on their faces. I knew they were thinking that I should be ashamed of myself. Third, I had three friends who had weight issues just like me and wanted to change their habits. So with a little help from my friends, I lost twenty pounds. And I'm not going to gain it back.

"We decided it was time to lose weight for two other reasons: our health and our appearances. Now, I know I'm doing everything I can to avoid diabetes and high blood pressure and other life-threatening diseases. And I think my hourglass shape is gorgeous! I look in the mirror and see a beautiful person. Watch out supermodels! Davanna Brown will meet up with you in the near future."

"I'd tell other teens a story like Davanna's," began Seth. "I'm a teenager who made decisions every day. Like when I got up in the morning, I'd decide whether to go to school or to skip class. When I walked into the door of the school, I'd decide whether to go down the hall or up the stairs. I'd also decide if I should eat lunch in the cafeteria or sneak out and go to the store next door.

"When I finally looked back at my ability to make decisions, I realized that everything I decided to do affected *me*. So in my bedroom one day I looked at myself in the mirror and asked, 'Seth, do you want to continue being called names because you're overweight? Aren't you tired of carrying around those twenty extra pounds as if you're carrying a twenty-pound baby? I decided it was time for *me* to change what I ate and work those pounds off my body frame.

"With help and support from my friends, I made a conscious decision not to be overweight. For years I was the guy whose only purpose in life was to tease other people. I thought I couldn't gain weight! Me being big, that would never happen! Then the pounds started to creep on. Before I knew it, I was overweight. Yes, I was fat.

"My weight affected my personality. Before, everyone who knew me knew that I was sarcastic and made fun of anyone and everyone who came my way. But when I became I overweight, my personality changed. Now people made fun of me. When I made a smart remark about someone, they'd turn around and respond with fat jokes. Back in the day, I teased this guy because his sneakers were torn. He said, 'You can laugh at my sneakers it you want to. But if your clothes ever catch on fire, don't forget you're supposed to stop, drop, and roll to smother the flames. But that would be a problem for you, because your butt is so fat. You'll have to stop, bounce, and roll. Do you get it? You'd bounce like a beach ball. Ha ha.'

"Then he laughed hysterically. The joke was on me and I was not used to it. Another time I teased this girl and told her that in her gym shorts she looked like a short dude. She said, 'I might look like a short dude, but when we go to Washington, D.C., for the White House tour, make sure your mother pays for two seats on the airplane, because your butt will need both of them. Okay!'

"People teased me with nothing but fat jokes. I thought, 'Oh hell no! I can't live in a fat body, it has ruined my image.'

"That was the first time I thought I might be overweight. I tried to see myself through the eyes of other people. I found out I was no longer the attractive funny guy. But that didn't stop me from eating all of the sweets in the house. I ate more, because I realized that I was going to be the one that other people teased. Yeah, I guess I felt sorry for myself.

"For years, I ran around confused about my weight like a hamster in a cage running inside a wheel. I never knew how to stop what I ate and how to lose the weight. I just ran from myself.

"Then I met Davanna, Maritza, and John, who were also overweight. We became friends. We were all smart, attractive, teased by other teens, and overweight. I guess subconsciously we all felt comfortable around each other. And we decided to work on it and change.

"Now I'm back to my ole attractive self, because I lost twenty pounds. I learned a valuable lesson. I have not forgotten how it felt to be teased when I was overweight. So I've stopped teasing others. Instead, I encourage them to eat healthy food and exercise. I tell them, 'If you're being teased, when you lose the weight you'll no longer be teased about it.'"

"My story is similar," said John. People used to call me tall, dark, and handsome. Ha ha."

"John, don't get it twisted!" said Davanna, looking at him like he was crazy. "You're tall and handsome, but not dark."

"Okay, calm down! Don't get so serious. Tall, dark, and handsome is an old cliché. I used to be physically active, until my mom got sick. After she passed away, my life spiraled down like a tornado cloud. I became depressed and didn't care about anything, including what I looked like. Food became my best friend, especially food that reminded me of my mom. The food stuck to my skinny bones. I used to be a tall, muscular guy with an athletic body. But I started to get round like an old beach ball. I lost control of what I put into my mouth. But I got my eating habits under control with help from my friends.

"I would tell other teenagers that they have the power to lose weight if they control the food they eat. They should throw away the junk food and sodas. They should start to read the labels on food before they just put it into their mouths. If the labels show a lot of sugar or sodium, which is salt, they might want to choose something else. I'd tell them to instead try foods that are good for their health.

"I know that sounds fake or corny, but it's true! There are foods that are good for our health just like there are foods that are bad for our health. If you have a craving for sweets, choose the ones that have nutrients in them, like fruit, lightly sweetened whole-grain cereals, and yogurt. Also, you can replace salt with different seasonings or flavors, like salt-free seasoning blends. Or pour lemon juice, lime juice, or flavored vinegars over food to bring out its natural taste.

"In the past we all ate all the pizza and fries we could swallow for lunch. Now we choose things like tacos with lettuce, tomatoes, and ground turkey. It might sound boring, but tacos are really good. You can put anything you want inside of them like beef, chicken, turkey, or beans.

"We also ate cake, cookies, and pie for dessert. We still eat dessert, but now we choose from a variety of fruits, low-fat puddings, and sorbets. We no longer crave foods that are not good for us, because we know better. The foods we eat are healthy. This is how we lost twenty pounds each. Some of us lost more than that. You can do it too.

"I'd tell others to just stick to healthy eating and begin to be physically active," John went on. "Take gossip walks, jog with a friend, shoot basketball, take a swim, or cheerlead. If you just keep doing that the weight will drop off you, like snow falling off a tree branch. I can't tell you where it goes, because you don't see puddles of weight around you on the ground. But it leaves your body."

"C'mon John, you know the weight leaves your body through sweat or through the, um, waste removal systems in your body," Davanna replied. "You know what I mean by that."

"What more could I add? " Maritza said. "I believe the three of you said it all. I guess I could say to other teens, 'You not only have the power to eat healthy, but you must. If not, you'll look like the old me before I lost twenty-two pounds. I was cute, and I was round. I looked like the fat blue exercise ball at the gym.' I'd tell them, 'Hey y'all, those donuts, coffee cakes, and hot pies you eat for breakfast are killing you. All of those foods contain large amounts of sugar that help you become overweight. Super-sized meals give you a super-sized body. Believe me, it's not pretty.'

"I used to eat all day. I ate a breakfast at home that my mom cooked, and then a breakfast at school. I had a lunch at school, then a pre-dinner at home, then dinner, and an after-dinner before bed. I ate as much a large grown man. Every meal I ate was a large portion too, and I never left a drop of food on my plate.

"I even ate when I wasn't hungry, because I was dealing with a lot of personal issues. Food was my best friend. As I kept eating, the pounds piled on. When kids called me fat names, I took a closer look at myself. There was one time a teen made several fat jokes about me. He said, 'Maritza looks like a fat hog. Maritza's butt is shaped like a large rump roast.'

"So I went home and looked in the mirror. That guy was right. I was that big fat girl he used in the jokes. I said, 'Oh my God, I'm fat!' I saw myself in a new way that day. I thought about a way to watch what I ate. I wanted to lose weight, but I couldn't figure it out alone.

"Then I hooked up with Davanna, John, and Seth. They understood my weight issues, because they had some of the same ones. They supported me and I supported them. I accomplished my weight goals because they understood me and supported me. I had carried around those twenty-two pounds with me for the past few years, and they had to be dropped. Changing my lifestyle wasn't easy, but it was damn sure worth it. Just look at me now. Now I'm a beautiful girl. I still have my caramel skin and busty boobs. But since I lost weight my thick bones and thunder thighs are gone, and I'm fine and I know it!

"Anyone can reach their weight goals by doing what we did. But you can't just change your diet or go to the gym once in a while. You have to make concrete lifestyle changes. Set aside some time to engage in daily physical activities such as aerobics, swimming, biking, jogging, or any other activity where you're moving around. Remember, you have to do it even when you don't want to."

Davanna said, "When I look at my picture before I lost weight and compare it to my picture now, I see how hard we worked at our changed lifestyles. I would show other teenagers these pictures so they could see the difference and understand how much hard work made a difference in our appearances. I'm not ashamed of showing them what I looked like or telling them how much I weighed."

Now the We Can't Weight Teens are no longer being teased or called names. They don't tease or call anyone else names either. They have more friends, their grades are better, and they participate more in school activities.

Remember the fat joke Davanna heard in the cafeteria? It went like this: "Fat kids don't run for student government. The only thing they run for at school is lunch."

Well, the We Can't Weight Teens have proved that joker wrong. Fat kids do run for student government. They also get elected.

The student body of Cedar Grove High elected all four friends as officers of the student government. Davanna is the president, Seth is the vice president, Maritza is the secretary, and John is the treasurer. As student government officers, the teens have started a health and wellness program at the school. They asked the student body to vote for more healthy food in the cafeteria, and the majority voted in favor. The teens have also worked to provide daily aerobics classes in the school gym in the mornings before classes start, and Zumba classes after school.

The student government officers also work with the school's guidance counselor to help provide peer counseling to overweight teens who want to lose weight. In an assembly, the We Can't Weight Teens told their weight-loss stories to the entire school. They did so hoping to help other students who needed support with their weight, healthy eating, and exercise.

The We Can't Weight Teens are popular in school. Davanna and Maritza get a lot of attention from guys, and the girls are after Seth and John. These are the same guys and girls who teased them when they were overweight. "Change some things about your lifestyle and a lot of other things change too," John says. "But I'm still me. I may be popular, but I'm still a computer geek."

John finally learned how to swim. To prove it, Malique had him swim from one side of the five-foot area to the other, and back. Then he had John tread water for one minute. John passed both tests and he is now allowed to swim in the deep end of the pool with the others. John meets Stacey at the pool on Saturdays. She volunteered to give him extra lessons, and has taught him several swimming strokes.

Davanna has taken private swimming lessons from Malique. She and John talk about swimming a lot.

Maritza became friends with Joshua, the physical trainer at the community center. She asked Joshua to meet with all four of the We Can't Weight Teens in the gym on Wednesdays before aerobics. Joshua agreed to help them tone up their muscles. His goal was to tighten up any loose skin that hung on their bodies after their weight loss. Skin stretches out on bodies that have been overweight over for a long period of time.

Joshua was especially interested in firming up Maritza's hourglass shape. Go figure!

As for Seth, he's still waiting to meet a special friend. But he gets his exercise daily and he eats right. And he knows the We Can't Weight Teens will always be there for him.

In the future, Davanna, Seth, John, and Maritza are hoping to travel across the United States to visit schools, youth groups, churches, synagogues, and clinics to talk to students who have weight issues. They want to create support groups for overweight teenagers like the one they started for each other.

Davanna, Seth, Maritza, and John say: "Good-bye for now. We'll talk again sometime soon. You might be hearing from us again soon to talk about the causes and effects of bullying."

# DISCUSSION QUESTIONS

- What should you do if you are being teased or bullied for being overweight?
- Should schools have a support system to address students who are either overweight or obese?
  - How should this support system work?
  - Who should be the members of the support system?
- What is the principal's role when a student is being teased or bullied because of his or her weight?
- Do you think overweight or obese teens are careful about the clothes they wear? If not, how could other teens talk to them about tight pants, miniskirts, or revealing shirts?
- What do you think about the self-esteem of overweight or obese teenagers? If it is not positive, how can teachers, parents, and peers support them?
- How did Ms. Lemon or Ms. Sussman support the We Can't Weight Teens? Did they help the teens with their self-esteem? How did they help the teens with their weight issues?
- What did you think about the parents? Talk about Davanna's, Maritza's, Seth's, and John's.
- Should teens that are not overweight or obese join support groups for overweight teens?

- Where do you think these support groups should be held? At schools, community centers, or clinics?
- Do you think parents of overweight or obese teens should be required to participate in the support groups?
- Should teens who have accomplished their weight goals be mentors for other overweight or obese teens?
- How did Davanna, Maritza, Seth, and John make you understand that being overweight or obese is a multicultural problem?

# ABOUT THE AUTHOR

Dr. Carol A. Brown is an administrator in a large urban school district in Massachusetts. At work and in the community, she provides guidance and support to overweight and obese teens. She holds a B.S. from Northeastern University in Boston, Massachusetts, a M.Ed. from Lesley University in Cambridge, Massachusetts, a CAGS from Bridgewater State University, and an Ed.D. from Nova Southeastern University in Miami, Florida. Dr. Brown lives in Boston Massachusetts.